ROBERT H. LUSTIG, M.D., is an internationally renowned pediatric endo-
crinologist who has spent the past 16 years treating childhood obesity and
studying the effects of sugar on the central nervous system, metabolism,
and disease. He is the Director of the Weight Assessment for Teen and Child
Health Program at UCSF Benioff Children's Hospital, a member of the
UCSF Center for Obesity Assessment, Study and Treatment, as well as a
member of the Obesity Task Force of The Endocrine Society.

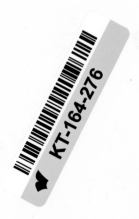

FAT CHANCE

●

The Bitter Truth
About Sugar

Robert H. Lustig, M.D.

FOURTH ESTATE • *London*

First published in Great Britain by
Fourth Estate
An imprint of HarperCollins*Publishers*
77–85 Fulham Palace Road
London W6 8JB
www.4thestate.co.uk

First published by Hudson Street Press, a member of the Penguin Group (USA) Inc.

1 3 5 7 9 10 8 6 4 2

A catalogue record for this book is
available from the British Library

ISBN 978-0-00-751412-0

Designed by Eve L. Kirch

Printed and bound in Great Britain by
Clays Ltd, St Ives plc

PUBLISHER'S NOTE
While the author has made every effort to provide accurate telephone numbers,
Internet addresses, and other contact information at the time of publication,
neither the publisher nor the author assumes any responsibility for errors, or for
changes that occur after publication. Further, the publisher does not have any
control over and does not assume any responsibility for author or third-party
websites or their content.

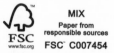

MIX
Paper from
responsible sources
FSC C007454

FSC™ is a non-profit international organisation established to promote
the responsible management of the world's forests. Products carrying the
FSC label are independently certified to assure consumers that they come
from forests that are managed to meet the social, economic and
ecological needs of present and future generations,
and other controlled sources.

Find out more about HarperCollins and the environment at
www.harpercollins.co.uk/green

This book is dedicated to all the obese patients worldwide who suffer daily, and the family members who suffer with them. The children who will not know a normal childhood, who will endure an inhuman existence, and will die a slow and early death. The parents who are engulfed by guilt. The unborn children, who are already imprisoned by changes in their brains and their bodies. But most of all, I dedicate this book to those of you who are or have been my patients; for it is you who taught me the science of your affliction. You also taught me more than medical school ever did or could; and that each life is valuable, precious, and worth saving. You maintained your dignity in the face of the most adverse circumstances imaginable. You shared with me your misery, and your joy in small victories. We cried and we laughed together. I hope I was of some service and comfort.

This book is my way of returning the favor.

This book is written only for those of you who eat food.
The rest of you are off the hook.

CONTENTS

Part IV. The "Real" Toxic Environment

Part V. The Personal Solution

Part VI. The Public Health Solution

INTRODUCTION:
Time to Think Outside the Box

"We just eat too damn much."

—Governor Tommy Thompson (R-Wisc.), U.S. Secretary of
Health and Human Services, *Today*, NBC, 2004

Indeed we do. That's it, thanks for buying this book, you've been a great audience, I'm outta here.

Well, that's what the U.S. government would have you believe. All the major U.S. governmental health agencies, the Centers for Disease Control (CDC), the U.S. Department of Agriculture (USDA), the Institute of Medicine (IOM), the National Institutes of Health (NIH), and the U.S. Surgeon General, say that obesity results from an energy imbalance: eating too many calories and not getting enough physical activity. And they are right—to a point. Are we eating more? Of course. Are we exercising less? No doubt. Despite knowing this, it hasn't made any difference in the rates of obesity or associated diseases. More to the point, how did this epidemic happen and in such a short interval of just thirty years? People say, "The food is there," and it is. But it was there before. People say, "The TV is there," and it is. But it was there before, and we didn't have this caloric catastrophe. There's more to this story, way more, and it's not pretty.

Everyone blames everyone else for what has happened. No way is it *their* fault. Big Food says it's a lack of activity due to computers and video games. The TV industry says it's our junk food diet. The Atkins people say it's too many carbohydrates; the Ornish people say it's too much fat. The juice people say it's the soda; the soda people say it's the juice. The schools say it's the parents; the parents say it's the schools. And since nothing is for sure, nothing is done. How do we reconcile all these opinions into a cohesive whole that actually makes sense and creates changes for the better for each individual and for all society? That's what this book is about.

Food is not tobacco, alcohol, or street drugs. Food is sustenance. Food is survival. Most important, food is pleasure. There are only two things that are more important than food: air and water. Shelter's a distant fourth. Food matters. Unfortunately, food now matters even more than it should. Food is beyond a necessity; it's also a commodity, and it has been reformulated to be an addictive substance.

This has many effects on our world: economically, politically, socially, and medically. There is a price to pay, and we're paying it now. We pay with our taxes, our insurance premiums, and our airline fares—nearly every bill we receive in the mail has an obesity surcharge that we underwrite. We pay in misery, worsening school scores, social devolution, and we pay in death. We pay for all of it, one way or another, because the current food environment we have created does not match our biochemistry, and this mismatch is at the heart of our medical, social, and financial crisis. Worse yet, there is no medicine for this. There is no edict, ordinance, legislation, tax, or law that can solve this alone. There is no quick fix, but the problem is resolvable if we know what's really going on—and if we really want to resolve it.

In his 2004 book *Food Fight*, Kelly Brownell of Yale University talks about obesity and the "toxic environment" we now live in, a euphemism for our collective bad behaviors. I am going a step further. I'm interested in whether there is something actually toxic, I mean *poisonous*, going on here. Even laboratory animal colonies have been getting fatter over the past twenty years!

Every good story needs a villain. While I am loath to reveal it this early in the book, I won't keep you in suspense. It's sugar—the Professor Moriarty of this story, a substance that now permeates nearly all food and drink worldwide. It's killing us . . . slowly, and I'll prove it. Every statement throughout this book is based on scientific study, historical fact, or recent statistics.

I'm a physician. We take an oath: *primum non nocere* (first do no harm). But there's a paradox in this statement: when you know the final disposition—that the outcome is going to be bad—then doing nothing is causing harm.

I certainly did not start out as an advocate. I wasn't looking for a fight. I didn't come to this controversy with a preconceived agenda. Indeed, I was fifteen years into my medical career before I stepped up to deal with obesity as an issue. Until 1995, like my medical colleagues, I did my best to avoid seeing obese patients. I had nothing to tell them except "it's your fault" and "eat less and exercise more." At that time, seeing an obese child with type 2 diabetes was an anomaly. Now it is an almost everyday occurrence. The problem of obesity is now inescapable in medical practice. You can't avoid it any more.

The concepts elaborated here didn't just wake me from sleep one day in a divine revelation. This book is the culmination of sixteen years of medical research, medical meetings, academic discourse with colleagues, journal clubs, policy analysis, and a whole lot of patient care. I have no conflict of interest in espousing the information here; I am not a pawn of the food industry or a mouthpiece for any organization. Unlike many authors addressing the devastation of obesity, I don't have a product line designed to enrich my bank account. I came by these views honestly and through rigorous data analysis. And the data are out there for everyone to examine. I'm just putting them together somewhat differently.

As a scientist, I have personally contributed to the understanding of the regulation of energy balance. As a pediatrician, I get to watch the interaction between genetics and environment that causes obesity play out in my examining room every day. And now, as a fledgling policy wonk, I have seen how the changes in our society have sprouted this global pandemic. It is this panoramic view that allows me to connect the dots for you, and they don't connect in the way you've been told.

To blame obesity on the obese is the easy answer, but it is the *wrong* answer. The current formulation of gluttony and sloth, diet and exercise, while accepted by virtually everyone, is based on faulty premises and myths that have taken hold in the world's consciousness. Obesity is not a behavioral aberration, a character flaw, or an error of commission. When we think about the ravages of obesity, our minds often go first to adults. But what about kids? One quarter of U.S children are now obese; even infants are tipping the scales! Children don't choose to be obese. They are victims, not perpetrators. Once you understand the science, you realize what applies to children also applies to grown-ups. I know what you're thinking: adults are responsible for their own choices and for the food they give their children. But are they?

An esteemed colleague involved in the obesity wars once said to me, "I don't care what's causing the obesity epidemic. I just want to know what to do about it." I respectfully disagree. In order to pull ourselves out of this ditch, we have to understand how we drove into it. Indeed, our current thinking is based on correlation, supposition, and conjecture. I wrote this book to persuade you, the reader, to take up this cause, for your own health and for our country's. However, you can't truly advocate for a cause unless you know what is going on. And you can't disagree with me until you know all the facts. And that means the science. After you've read this book, if you think it's a crock or that I'm a crank, tell me. I want to know. In fact, I'll make a promise to you right now: there is not one statement made in this entire book that can't be backed up by hard science. My reputation in the field is built on the science. It's also my protection against those who would try to discredit me, including the food industry and, as you will see, the federal government. Indeed, it's the only reason I haven't been discredited yet. And I won't be, because I stick to the science. Now and forever.

However, in four places in the book, I let my imagination run wild. I will try to explain how obesity fits within the process of evolution, how our evolutionary biochemistry works to keep us alive, and finally how our food environment has altered that biochemistry to promote this global catastrophe. These fits of speculation will carry the section heading "Deconstructing Darwin."

This book is targeted at the patients who suffer, the doctors who suffer along with them, the U.S. electorate who pays for this debacle, the politicians who must take up arms to dig us out of the mess that has been created out of our economy and our health, and the rest of the world, so they don't make the same mistakes (although they already have).

In part 1 of this book, I will challenge some of the theories you're used to hearing in the media, and indeed from the medical profession. Parts 2 and 3 will focus on the science of obesity, and how the body deals with energy burning versus storage. No, you don't need to be a biology or medical expert to understand the science. I've worked hard to reduce it down to its essence, and to keep it interesting, light, and accessible. In part 2, I'll also explain how your brain has developed, evolutionarily and *in utero*, to thwart your attempts at dieting. You truly are hormonal when it comes to the foods you crave, just not in the ways you think. Part 3 will elaborate on the science of fat tissue, and when and how it can make you sick. In part 4, I will prove that our current environment is indeed "toxic." I will show how the "American diet," which is now the "industrial global diet," is killing us . . . slowly. I will identify the poison and the antidotes, why those antidotes work, and why they've been added to or removed from our diet for the food industry's purposes. Part 5 elaborates what you, as an individual, can do to protect yourself and your family by changing your "personal environment." Finally, in part 6, I argue that governments around the world have been co-opted by the food industry, and I will outline how they must instead partner with the populace and exert influence over the food industry to stop the obesity pandemic before we all reach the medical and financial Armageddon now within sight.

PART I

The Greatest Story Ever Sold

Chapter 1

A Fallacy of Biblical Proportion

———————•———————

Juan, a 100-pound six-year-old Latino boy whose mother is a non-English-speaking farm worker from Salinas, California, comes to my clinic in 2003. He is wider than he is tall. I ask the mother in my broken Spanish, "I don't care what your kid eats, tell me what he drinks." No soda, but a gallon of orange juice per day. On calories alone, this accounts for 112 pounds per year of body fat. Of course, some of that is burned off, and it might influence total food intake. I explain to the mother, "*La fruta es buena, el jugo es malo* (the fruit is good, the juice is bad). Eat the fruit, don't drink the juice." She asks, "Then why does WIC [Women, Infants, and Children, a government entitlement program for the poor run by the U.S. Department of Agriculture] give it to us?"

One kid, one mother, one question, my life was changed—and the need for this book was born. Why *does* WIC give it to them? There is real science behind our worldwide obesity catastrophe. And science should drive policy, but as you will see, the politics get in the way. This is the most complex issue facing the human race this side of the Middle East conflict. And it has become incrementally more complicated over time, with multitudes of stakeholders with set agendas, and bigger than the individual parties involved. Devoid of simple solutions, it has destroyed families and claimed the lives of countless people.

You can't pick up a newspaper or log on to the Internet without seeing some new statistic on the obesity pandemic. It's all obesity, all the time. And how many of them have something good to report? You can bet that any tabloid headline is about one of two things—either the statistics are getting worse or another obesity drug was denied or withdrawn by the Food and Drug Administration. I'm sure you're sick of it. I know I am. And weight loss has turned into a blood sport—just tune in to *The Biggest Loser*.

In 2001, *Newsweek* reported that six million kids in America were seriously overweight. We have tripled that number in a decade, and the numbers are now surpassing twenty million. Yet for all the media attention, visibility, discussion, and weight loss programs, even Michelle Obama can't put the genie back in the bottle.

While we're getting fatter, we're also getting sicker. Our risk for illness is increasing faster than the increase in obesity. Indeed, the cluster of chronic metabolic diseases termed metabolic syndrome—which includes obesity, type 2 diabetes, hypertension (high blood pressure), lipid (blood fat) disorders, and cardiovascular (heart) disease—is snowballing by leaps and bounds. And then there are the other obesity-associated metabolic diseases, such as nonalcoholic fatty liver disease, kidney disease, and polycystic ovarian syndrome. Add to that the other comorbidities (related medical conditions) associated with obesity, such as orthopedic problems, sleep apnea, gallstones, and depression, and the medical devastation associated with the obesity pandemic is staggering. Every one of these diseases has become more prevalent over the past thirty years. What's more, all of them are now found in children as young as five years old. We even have an epidemic of obese six-month-olds![1]

The human damage in this scourge of metabolic syndrome is showing. In 2005 one study showed that despite the increased availability of medical care, our children will be the first generation of Americans who will die earlier than their forebears.[2] The study placed the blame squarely on the obesity epidemic. In the United States, quality-adjusted life years lost to obesity have more than doubled from 1993 to 2008. Emergency rooms are taking care of forty-year-old heart attack victims. Teens with type 2 diabetes used to be unheard of; now they are one third of all new diagnoses of diabetes. In the United States alone, 160,000 bariatric surgeries (to reduce the size of the stomach) are performed per year, at an average cost of $30,000 per surgery. Over 40 percent of death certificates now list diabetes as the cause of death, up from 13 percent twenty years ago.

The loss in American productivity due to time off from work is staggering, the waste in medical expenditures ($147 billion per year) is breaking the bank, and this amount is predicted to increase to $192 billion by the end of the decade. Guess what? There's no money to pay for it all. The Affordable Care Act (ACA, or "Obamacare") is going to put thirty-two million sick people on the insurance rolls by 2019. The president says we'll make up for the costs in savings from preventative care. However, it is unlikely to improve our health in any significant way, as there are no provisions for the prevention of chronic disease, most notably those that attend obesity. How do you prevent all the ravages of chronic metabolic disease when we bust the scales and when the statistics show no sign of improvement? It's often been said that we wouldn't need health care reform if we had obesity reform.

It would be one thing if obesity were an isolated problem in America, but it's happening everywhere. The obesity pandemic has expanded the world's collective waistline. The World Health Organization (WHO) has shown that the percentage of obese humans globally has doubled in the past twenty-eight years. In fact, obesity's contribution to the burden of chronic disease has been equal to if not greater than that of smoking. Even people in developing countries are obese. After only one decade, there are now 30 percent more people who are obese than are undernourished worldwide. The WHO reported in 2008 that approximately 1.5 billion adults were overweight and at least 400 million were obese globally[3]; these numbers are projected to reach about 2.3 billion and 700 million, respectively, by 2015. In September 2011 the UN General Assembly declared that non-communicable diseases (diabetes, cancer, and heart disease) are now a greater threat to world health than are infectious diseases, including in the developing world (see chapter 22). Is the whole world now composed of gluttons and sloths? Over the next fifteen years, these diseases will cost low- and middle-income countries more than $7 trillion.[4] People are dying earlier, and national economies are losing billions of dollars in lost productivity while governments pay for the medical expenditures. Millions of families end up in poverty, guaranteeing that the cycle will not be reversed.

For the 55 percent of adults who are overweight or obese, listen up. I'm talking to *you*, at a doctor-to-patient level, at a person-to-person level. Obesity is not an automatic death sentence. A full 20 percent of morbidly obese persons are metabolically healthy and have normal life spans.[5] As for the other 80 percent, you don't have to be in poor health; everyone has it within his reach to improve his health and regain those years the actuaries say will be lost. But success in doing so depends on identifying the cause of the problem, assessing your metabolic risk, and changing your biochemistry. Okay, full disclosure: despite your best efforts, you may never lose your stubborn subcutaneous fat (the fat that pads your thighs and derrière). And if you do, you'll gain it back in short order—unless you become a gym rat, because vigorous exercise is the only rational way to prevent weight regain (see chapter 13). In fact, if you lose meaningful amounts of subcutaneous fat and keep it off for more than a year, I'll be shocked. Pleasantly so, but shocked nonetheless.

For the 45 percent of adults who are normal weight, pay attention. You either sneer at or pity the other 55 percent of your brethren who take up two seats on the bus. You look down on them as weak, overindulgent, and lazy. You resent them, and you show it financially and socially. You're indignant that they cost you money. And you think you're out of the woods and home free. You've been told that you'll live a long and happy life. Whatever you're doing, it must be right. For those of you who are "naturally" thin, you've been told that you have great genes and can consume all the soft drinks and Twinkies you want without gaining a pound or getting sick. Would that it were true. A few years ago, you were the majority of Americans. Now you're the minority. And you're losing your percentage year by year.

This means that many of you are flipping—that is, gaining weight and going over to the dark side. Indeed, current projections suggest that by 2030, the United States will be 65 percent overweight and 165 million American adults will be obese.[6] The 2008 movie *Wall-E* is a prophecy: that's where we're all headed. We'll all be so fat, we'll have to ride around on little scooters, just like at Walmart. And as you get older, your risk for gaining weight keeps going up. Your genes won't change, but your biochemistry will. So, if you're flipping (which more and more of you are), something must be sending you over to the "dark side." And if that's not your fate, it will be that of your children. Nobody knows this better than I, because I take care of those children every day.

Here's the kicker. Being thin is not a safeguard against metabolic disease or early death. Up to 40 percent of normal-weight individuals harbor insulin resistance—a sign of chronic metabolic disease—which will likely shorten their life expectancy. Of those, 20 percent demonstrate liver fat on an MRI of the abdomen (see chapter 8).[7] Liver fat, irrespective of body fat, has been shown to be a major risk factor in the development of diabetes. You think you're safe? You are *so* screwed. And you don't even know it.

The overriding thesis of this book is that your fat is not your fate—provided you don't surrender. Because people don't die of obesity per se. They die of what happens to their organs. On the death certificate, the medical examiner doesn't write down "obesity"; instead it's "heart attack," "heart failure," "stroke," "diabetes," "cancer," "dementia," or "cirrhosis of the liver." These are diseases that "travel" with obesity. They are all chronic metabolic diseases. But normal-weight people die of these as well. *That's the point.* It's not the obesity. The obesity is not the *cause* of chronic metabolic disease. It's a *marker* of chronic metabolic disease, otherwise known as metabolic syndrome. And it's metabolic syndrome that will kill you. Understanding this distinction is crucial to improving your health, no matter your size. Obesity and metabolic syndrome overlap, but they are different. Obesity doesn't kill. Metabolic syndrome kills. Although they travel together, one doesn't cause the other. But then, what causes obesity? And what causes metabolic syndrome? And what can you do about each? Read on.

I wrote this book to help you and your kids get healthy and improve your quality of life, increase your productivity, and reduce the world's waste of medical resources. If you get thin in the process, great. But if that's what you expect, go find your own diet guru, and good luck with that. Want to get healthier? Want to get happier? Want to get smarter? It's your visceral (around your abdominal organs) fat and hepatic (liver) fat that's keeping you down. And getting rid of visceral fat is not as hard as you might think. This is the more metabolically active fat, and there's plenty you can do to shrink it.

A proverb says, "A journey of a thousand miles begins with a single step." This book is a journey into the workings of the body. It is a journey into the biochemistry of our brains and our fat cells. It is a journey into evolution, the mismatch between our environment and our biochemistry. And it is a journey into the world of business and politics, too. This journey starts with a single but very large step, in which we abandon our current thinking of obesity by challenging the age-old dogma "*a calorie is a calorie.*"

Chapter 2

A Calorie Is a Calorie—or Is It?

———————•———————

"If folks want to maintain a healthy weight, they have to be
sensitive to the calories in and calories out . . . Not every calorie
is the same."

—Governor Tom Vilsack (D-Iowa), U.S. Secretary of Agriculture,
upon release of the 2010 Dietary Guidelines, January 13, 2011

Wait a second. If people have to be sensitive to calories in and out, then
why aren't calories the same? Does anyone see the contradiction
here? This was the first time that any government official had even remotely
hinted that calories might not be interchangeable, and it was buried in this
cryptic double-speak.

Everyone is a dietitian. Everyone thinks he or she understands
obesity. Believe it or not, this is one of the harder medical conditions to
comprehend. Why? Obesity is a combination of several factors: physics,
biochemistry, endocrinology, neuroscience, psychology, sociology, and
environmental health, all rolled up into one problem. The factors that
drive the obesity pandemic are almost as myriad as the number of people
who suffer from it.

The Venus Von Willendorf is an eleven-inch statue carbon-dated to
22,000 BCE that was unearthed in Austria in 1908 (see figure 2.1). It depicts
the torso of a morbidly obese adult woman. This shows us that the ancients
knew about obesity long before they knew about fast food. There are other
ways to gain weight aside from potato chips and pizza, soda and suds. The
medical literature lists at least thirty diagnoses that include obesity as a
symptom. These include problems of the brain, liver, and adipose (fat) tis-

sue; genetic disorders; various hormonal imbalances; and the effects of certain medications.

But none of these medical causes explain what's happened to the
world's population over the last thirty years. Until 1980, statistically only 15
percent of the adult population had a body mass index—or BMI, an indicator of body fatness that is calculated from a person's weight and height—
above the eighty-fifth percentile, indicating either overweight or obesity.
Now that statistic is 55 percent. And by 2030 it's expected to be 65 percent.[1]
Something's happened in the last thirty years, but what?

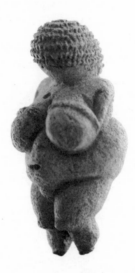

Fig. 2.1. A Venus FatTrap. The Venus von Willendorf is an 11-cm-high statuette
of a female that carbon-dates to between 24,000 and 22,000 BCE. It was discovered in 1908 in Austria, and is on display in the Naturhistorisches Museum in
Vienna. It shows that obesity is as old as man (or woman) himself.

The First Law

In order to understand obesity, and energy balance in general, we must acquaint
ourselves with the first law of thermodynamics, which states, "The total energy
inside a closed system remains constant." For you math and science geeks:

$$U = Q - W$$

where U is the internal energy of a system, Q is the heat supplied by the system, and W is the work done by the system. Work and heat are due to processes that either add or subtract energy; when work = heat, the internal energy stays constant. The first law is a *law*. It is elegant and airtight. If you don't like it, file a grievance with Sir Isaac Newton. I subscribe to the first law. The basis for our current understanding of the causes and consequences of the obesity pandemic lies not with the first law itself, but rather in how you interpret it, for, as with all laws, there is plenty of room for alternative interpretations.

The prevailing wisdom on the first law can be summed up by one widely held dogma: *a calorie is a calorie*. That is, to maintain energy balance and body weight (the U in the equation), one calorie eaten (the Q) must be offset by one calorie burned (the W). The calorie eaten can come from anywhere, from meat to vegetables to cheesecake. The calorie burned can go to anywhere, from sleeping to watching TV to vigorous exercise. And from this dogma comes the standard and widely held interpretation of the first law: "If you eat it, you had better burn it, or you will store it." In this interpretation, the behaviors of increased energy intake and decreased energy expenditure are primary (and presumably learned); therefore, the weight gained is a secondary result. Thus, obesity is routinely thought to be the natural consequence of these "aberrant behaviors." As you will see hereafter, virtually all the stakeholders in the obesity pandemic have signed up on the side of personal responsibility.

The Seating Chart at the Table of Blame

The Head of the Table: The Gluttons and the Sloths

Personal responsibility occupies the biggest seat at the Table of Blame. The common assumption in obesity hinges on its being a personal choice: We control what we eat and how much we exercise. If you are obese, it must be because you chose to either eat more, exercise less, or both. Over the past twenty-five years, various government agencies have accumulated ample evidence of the increased caloric intake during that time frame, both in children and in adults. During this time, the CDC has documented that Americans have increased their caloric consumption by an extra 187 calories per day for men, 335 calories per day for women. The behaviors associated with the rise in obesity include increased consumption of sugar-sweetened beverages and decreased consumption of whole fruits, vegetables, and other sources of dietary fiber. On a societal level, obesity is also associated with less breastfeeding, skipped breakfasts, fewer family meals, and more fast food dining. Alternatively, a wealth of evidence supports a role for decreased physical activity and increased "screen time" (TV, computers, video games, and texting) in causing obesity.

It is from this perception of choice that we derive our current societal mantras around obesity: gluttony and sloth, two of the original "seven deadly sins." I should note here that people exhibiting the other five deadly sins (greed, pride, lust, envy, and wrath) have gotten a pass in the press and in society as a whole. They are frequently extolled in the media—just watch the reality shows *The Apprentice* (envy, greed, pride, wrath—"You're Fired!"), *Millionaire Matchmaker* (lust, greed, pride), or *Jersey Shore* (all known sins and then some).

We've found absolution for nearly every vice and sin we can commit, except for these two. They continue to defy our society's ability to forgive. This despite the fact that 55 percent of Americans are either overweight or obese. Thin people are now in the minority, yet our culture continues to punish the majority. The average woman in the United States wears a size 14, yet many stores do not carry anything above a size 10. Although many women's clothing stores now have "vanity sizes" (what was a size 10 in 1950 is now labeled a size 6), a large percentage of the population still can't find anything on the rack. Approximately ten years ago in San Francisco, a billboard advertising the local 24-Hour Fitness health club depicted an extraterrestrial with the tag line "When they come, they'll eat the fat ones first."

Our society continues to glorify thinness even though it appears to be less achievable every year. Those of us who are overweight or obese are immediately assumed to be gluttons and/or sloths. The obese are passed over for employment because it's assumed they'll be as lazy on the job as they are in caring for their bodies. They are among the last groups about which you can still make pejorative comments in public. From this condemnation, it's a quick jump to the determination that obese people became so due to a behavioral defect. This formulation serves many purposes. It certainly justifies society's desire to place blame.

Even the obese have bought into the thesis of personal responsibility (see chapter 20). They would prefer to be portrayed as "perpetrator" rather than "victim." If you're a perpetrator, you maintain control and make your own choices, which is more hopeful than the alternative. If, instead, you're a victim, you have no power, obesity is your fate, and there is no hope. You're doomed, which is far more depressing. Finally, "personal responsibility" serves as the cornerstone of both the government's and the insurance companies' restriction of obesity care delivery.

Seat 2: The Health Insurance Industry

Much of the public views doctors as moneymaking mountebanks who care less for their patients than for their wallets. Well, we lose money on every patient we see. While our hospital's general pediatric health insurance reimbursement averages 37.5 cents on the dollar (a pittance), our pediatric obesity clinic collects only 29.0 cents per dollar billed. The reason for this? The health insurance industry refuses to pay for obesity services, saying, "Obesity is a behavior, a flaw in your character, a psychological aberration. And we don't pay for behavior." This is the reason that, despite having enough business many times over, childhood obesity clinics and treatment programs are closing across the country. The insurance industry has decided that obesity is a lifestyle choice; therefore, it won't pay. And when insurance companies do pay, they pay the absolute minimum.

The insurance industry hates this obesity epidemic almost as much as we doctors do. They are hunkering down for a long siege. Why do they continue to deny reimbursement for obesity services? Because if they paid for all the services required by today's pandemic, it would break their piggybank. Instead, they keep plugging holes in the dike by ascribing blame to the individual. They know that if they ever admit that obesity is the fault of no one person, the waters will engulf them all.

Seat 3: The Medical Profession

Twenty years ago, obesity was a social issue, not a medical one. At the beginning of my career, a colleague in pediatric endocrinology (the study of hormones in children) would send a form letter to the parents of children referred for obesity that read, "Dear parent, thank you for your interest in our pediatric endocrinology division. Your child has been referred for obesity. Obesity is a problem of nutrition and activity, not one of endocrinology. We suggest that you seek general advice from your child's pediatrician." And despite the undeniable onslaught of patients referred, many of my colleagues still feel this way.

As the problems have soared and the research dollars have poured in, the American Diabetes Association (ADA), the American Heart Association (AHA), and countless others professional organizations have devoted a substantial portion of their agendas to the obesity pandemic. The standard mantra espoused by the medical establishment is, "Lifestyle causes obesity, and obesity causes metabolic syndrome." We doctors recognize our role in mitigating the negative effects of obesity. But, again, for most physicians, the behaviors come first. The fault still lies with the patient.

Seat 4: The Obesity Profiteers

They say, "You're weak. You've failed. Let us help you." They profess to have the answer for your obesity problem and are peddling one solution or another. They are the obesity profiteers, and they represent large and vast industries, most of which are ostensibly trying to "do the right thing," while making a fortune in the process. We have the otherwise reputable peer-group weight-loss programs such as Weight Watchers and Jenny Craig, which strongly recommend the option of buying their trademarked cuisine (often loaded with sodium) to bolster profits. There are the diet supplement people such as Nutri-System, who demand that you purchase their food if you want to see results. Gym programs such as Curves and 24-Hour Fitness charge initiation and renewal fees for membership. Then there are the companies that make home exercise equipment. Their late-night infomercials invariably show a buff guy stretching a rubber band with the implicit message, "You can look like this if you stretch a rubber band." And then we have the "obesity authors" (gee, I'm one now!). Some are M.D.s, some Ph.D.s, some journalists, some pop culture phenomena, and some charlatans (none of which is mutually exclusive). All profess to have the answer to your obesity problem, peddling one diet or another. A few of these authors have developed corporations that want to sell you their food line, such as Atkins or the Zone. And each provides just enough science and nuggets of truth to hook the public.

Some weight-loss doctors and clinics peddle prescription appetite suppressants or other weight-loss remedies—all of which are paid for out of pocket. Some of these doctors are reputable and brilliant academics at medical universities who are trying to save people's lives while studying the physiology of obesity. Some are surgeons who perform liposuction for cosmetic purposes and bariatric surgery for metabolic and cardiac rescue. But some of them are "cut-and-run" surgeons operating out of small airplanes and flying around to little towns to perform quickie lap-band surgeries or gastric bypasses. They take their victims' money, have no quality control, never see the patient in follow-up, and sometimes leave medical catastrophes in their wake.

While the insurance companies refuse to shell out funds for this problem, the research money is pouring in. The pharmaceutical industry has spent a lot of money to come up with the "obesity blockbuster," that magic bullet that will work long-term and for everyone. But that's a pipe dream because, first, obesity isn't one disease, it's many; second, our bodies have many redundant pathways to maintain our critical energy balance, so one drug can't possibly be effective for everyone; and third, there's no one drug that will treat metabolic syndrome (see chapter 19).

Each of these people and industries have one thing in common: they are trying to make a buck off the misfortunes of the obese, to the tune of $117 billion a year. And they're all charging retail. Out of pocket, cash on the barrelhead. No insurance reimbursements here. No discounts. In case you hadn't noticed, the obese will do *anything* not to be obese, even throw their money away on "get-thin-quick" schemes. That's why these industries are the obesity profiteers. Do any of their "solutions" work? Fat chance. If you just did what they told you, the fat would magically disappear. If it fails, it's your fault—you must have been noncompliant! Yet another reason for the obese to be depressed. Think about it—if any of these books, diets, or programs actually worked for the entire population, there would be only one. The person who makes this discovery will likely win the Nobel Prize, move to a mansion in Tahiti, and be featured on *Lifestyles of the Rich and Famous*.

Seat 5: The Fat Activists

There's nothing socially or medically wrong with being fit and fat; you're doing better than the people out there who are thin and sedentary. But there is something medically wrong with being fat and *sick*. Especially if you're suffering metabolically, which 80 percent of obese people are. If you fall into this category, you are costing society money in caring for your metabolic illnesses, reducing productivity, and clogging up (and bringing down) the health care system. Not to mention digging yourself an early grave! The vocal proponents for the political and social rights of the obese, primarily the National Association to Advance Fat Acceptance (NAAFA), say, "Being fat is a badge of honor. Be fit and fat, be fat and proud." No victimization here. And I agree. But NAAFA is also opposed to academic obesity research where its primary goal is weight loss—because why would you investigate a condition that is totally normal? They don't think attention should be paid to how much kids weigh. This is puzzling to me. There is something highly paradoxical about enabling your child to be fat and sick. The majority of obese kids will be diabetic and cardiac cripples by the time they're fifty. The science and research that NAAFA's policy would seem to exclude are critical to studying this epidemic and determining what we can do about it. It's my job as a pediatrician to protect these kids from such misguided thinking.

Seat 6: The Commercial Food Industry

The commercial food industry responds to the obesity pandemic with two mantras. First, "Everyone is responsible for what goes into his or her mouth." Is that true? What goes into our mouths depends on two things: selectivity and access. Second, "Any food can be part of a balanced diet." True but irrelevant because, thanks to the food industry, we don't have a balanced diet, and they're the ones that unbalanced it. They are a major instigator of the obesity pandemic through both their actions and the kind of rhetoric they use to justify those actions. Corporations repeatedly say one thing, yet do another. McDonald's now advertises a healthier menu, with commercials featuring slim people in exercise clothes eating salads. However, the vast majority of people entering McDonald's, even if they come in with the idea of eating a salad, instead order a Big Mac and fries. And McDonald's is well aware of this. Its recent billboard campaign, "Crafted for Your Craving," says all you need to know. Carl's Jr.'s promotion of the "Western Bacon Six Dollar Burger," which has a whopping 1,030 calories and 55 grams of fat, generally depicts fit and attractive people consuming the company's fare with relish. Do you really think they would continue to be thin if they ate this on a regular basis?

Food has become a commodity (see chapter 21), with foodstuffs that can be stored being traded on the various commodities exchanges. Speculators can corner the market on anything, from pork bellies to orange juice, by betting how much the price will rise and fall. And it's because individual foods are treated as commodities that the downstream effects of changes in the food supply, and subsequently food prices, are being felt worldwide (see chapter 21). Cheap food means political stability. There is an imperative to keep food highly available and the prices as low as possible. Everyone is *for* cheap food. The United States spends 7 percent of its gross domestic product (GDP) on food, which allows the populace to buy more DVDs and iPads and take more vacations. But cheaper food, loaded with preservatives for longer shelf life, costs you on the tail end, and way more than all your gadgets and vacations put together (with interest).

Seat 7: The Federal Government

Our government is extraordinarily conflicted about where it should stand on the obesity pandemic. In 2003, former U.S. surgeon general Richard Carmona stated that obesity was an issue of national security, a stance that current surgeon general Regina Benjamin has upheld (despite the fact that she herself is obese) and one to which the U.S. Army has signed on. The public health branches of the government tell us that we eat too much and exercise too little. Mrs. Obama's Let's Move! campaign centers on the idea that childhood obesity can be battled by planting school vegetable gardens, encouraging kids to get out and exercise, and remaking the School Nutrition Act. *All necessary, but not sufficient.*

The U.S. government does everything it can to keep food cheap (see chapter 16). The USDA has chosen not to accept any responsibility for its role in the obesity pandemic, continuing to market our Western diet around the world. The Farm Bill (see chapter 21) maintains food subsidies to keep farmers employed and growing more crops. The growers make their profits on volume. The food processors make big markups and pass them along to the consumer. And the USDA subsidizes food entitlement programs to the poor, such as the Supplemental Nutrition Assistance Program (SNAP, formerly known as food stamps) and the Women, Infants, and Children nutrition program (or WIC, which supplies low-income infants and their mothers with food and health care), to keep them alive and complacent. Until 2007, WIC bowed to the pressure of food lobbyists. The foodstuffs provided were largely unhealthy, and included white bread and high-sugar juices.

The "Food Pyramid," the federal nutrition guide released in 1974 (see figure 2.2a) and revised every five years, culminating with "MyPyramid" in 2005, was never based on science. Indeed it was top and bottom heavy—hardly a pyramid. In response to calls for revision from many in the medical community, the Food Pyramid was deep-sixed in 2011. "MyPyramid" has now

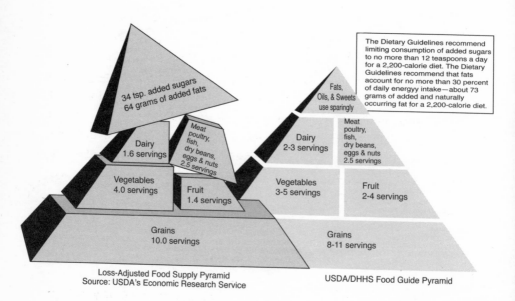

The Dietary Guidelines recommend limiting consumption of added sugars to no more than 12 teaspoons a day for a 2,200-calorie diet. The Dietary Guidelines recommend that fats account for no more than 30 percent of daily energyy intake—about 73 grams of added and naturally occurring fat for a 2,200-calorie diet.

34 tsp. added sugars
64 grams of added fats

Dairy
1.6 servings

Meat poultry, fish, dry beans, eggs & nuts
2.5 servings

Vegetables
4.0 servings

Fruit
1.4 servings

Grains
10.0 servings

Loss-Adjusted Food Supply Pyramid
Source: USDA's Economic Research Service

Fats, Oils, & Sweets use sparingly

Meat poultry, fish, dry beans, eggs & nuts
2.5 servings

Dairy
2-3 servings

Vegetables
3-5 servings

Fruit
2-4 servings

Grains
8-11 servings

USDA/DHHS Food Guide Pyramid

Fig. 2.2a. The Ancient Pyramids. The traditional USDA Food Pyramid, circa 2005, which advised us to eat more grains and less fat and sugar. Alongside it, what Americans actually ate—more like an hourglass than a pyramid.

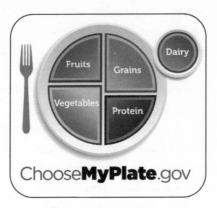

Fig. 2.2b. The Modern Merry-Go-Round. Under pressure from consumer groups and in response to the emerging science, the Pyramid was relegated to ancient history, and MyPlate was adopted by the USDA in 2011. MyPlate advises us to eat approximately half a plate of vegetables or fruits, one quarter fiber-containing starch such as brown rice, and one quarter protein, preferably low-fat. It's too early to tell if this change will have any effect on American eating habits.

morphed into "MyPlate" (see figure 2.2b). The most recent guidance from the Dietary Guidelines Advisory Committee (DGAC), released in 2010, says that obesity is a problem (shocker) so we should all eat less fat, sugar, and salt. We're all supposed to eat more fruits and vegetables, and less of everything else. This is stating the obvious. Don't we already know this? Eat less? How? If we *could* eat less, there wouldn't be an obesity pandemic. But we can't.

Each of the stakeholders in the obesity pandemic is singing the same tune: "Your obesity is your personal responsibility, it's your fault, and you've failed." And all these accusations are a variation on a theme based on one unflappable dogma: *a calorie is a calorie.*

Calories Don't Count If . . .

The clues are all around us as to what's really happened. It's time to look at where those extra calories went, because it is in these data that we will find the answer to the obesity dilemma.

There are three problems with "*a calorie is a calorie.*"

First, there is no way anyone could actually burn off the calories supplied by our current food supply. A chocolate chip cookie has the equivalent calories of twenty minutes of jogging, and working off a Big Mac would require *four hours* of biking. But, wait! Olympic swimmer Michael Phelps eats 12,000 calories a day and burns them off, right? If this were the case for all of us, diet and exercise should work—you'd burn more than you ate and lose weight (see chapter 13). And diet drugs should work—you take the drug, eat or absorb less, and lose the pounds. Except the meds don't deliver on their promises. They work for a brief period, and then patients reach a plateau in weight loss (see chapter 4).[2] Why? Do the patients stop taking the pills? No. So why do the medications stop working? The answer: because the body is smarter than the brain is. Energy expenditure is reduced to meet the decreased energy intake. So a calorie is *not* really a calorie, because your caloric output is controlled by your body and is dependent on the quantity *and* the quality of the calories ingested.

Second, if *a calorie is a calorie,* then all fats would be the same because they'd each release 9.0 calories per gram of energy when burned. But they're not all the same. There are good fats (which have valuable properties, such as being anti-inflammatory) and bad fats (which can cause heart disease and fatty liver disease; see chapter 10). Likewise, all proteins and amino acids should be the same, since they release 4.1 calories per gram of energy when burned. Except that we have high-quality protein (such as egg protein), which may reduce appetite, and we have low-quality protein (hamburger meat), which is full of branched-chain amino acids (see chapter 9), which has been associated with insulin resistance and metabolic syndrome.[3] Finally, all carbohydrates should be the same, since they also release 4.1 calories per gram of energy when burned. But they're not. A closer look at the specific breakdown of the carbohydrate data reveals something interesting. There are two classes of carbohydrate: starch and sugar. Starch is made up of glucose only, which is not very sweet and which every cell in the body can use for energy. Although there are several other "sugars" (glucose, galactose, maltose, and lactose), when I talk about sugar here (and in the rest of this book), I am talking about the "sweet" stuff, sucrose and high-fructose corn syrup, which both contain the molecule fructose. Fructose is *very* sweet and is inevitably metabolized to fat (see chapter 11). It is the primary (although not the sole) villain, the Darth Vader of the Empire, beckoning you to the dark side in this sordid tale.

The third problem with *"a calorie is a calorie"* is illustrated by the U.S. secretary of health and human services Tommy Thompson's admonishment in 2004 that we're "eating too damn much," would suggest that we're eating more of everything. But we're not eating more of *everything*. We're eating more of some things and less of others. And it is in those "some things" that we will find our answer to the obesity pandemic. The U.S. Department of Agriculture keeps track of nutrient disappearance. These data show that *total consumption* of protein and fat remained relatively constant as the obesity pandemic accelerated. Yet, due to the "low-fat" directives in the 1980s of the AMA, AHA, and USDA, the intake of fat declined as a *percentage of total calories* (from 40 percent to 30 percent). Protein intake remained relatively constant at 15 percent. But if total calories increased, yet the total consumption of fat was unchanged, that means something had to go up. Examination of the carbohydrate data provides the answer. As a percentage of total caloric intake, the intake of carbohydrates increased from 40 percent to 55 percent.[4] While it's true we are eating more of both classes of carbohydrate (starch and sugar), our total starch intake has risen from just 49 to 51 percent of calories. Yet our fructose intake has increased from 8 percent to 12 percent to, in some cases (especially among children), 15 percent of total calories. So it stands to reason that what we're eating more of is sugar, specifically fructose. Our consumption of fructose has doubled in the past thirty years and has increased sixfold in the last century. The answer to our global dilemma lies in understanding the causes and effects of this change in our diet.

There's one lesson to conclude from these three contradictions to the current dogma. *A calorie is not a calorie*. Rather, perhaps the dogma should be restated thus: a calorie burned *is* a calorie burned, but a calorie eaten *is not* a calorie eaten. And therein lies the key to understanding the obesity pandemic. The quality of what we eat determines the quantity. It also determines our desire to burn it. And personal responsibility? Just another urban myth to be busted by real science.

Chapter 3

Personal Responsibility
versus the Obese Six-Month-Old

———————•———————

Sienna is a one-year-old girl who weighs 44 pounds. She was 10 pounds at birth and was delivered by caesarean section due to her size. Her mother is not obese, but her father is overweight. Her mother tested negative for diabetes during the pregnancy. Since birth, Sienna has had an incredible appetite. Her mother could not breastfeed her because she could not keep up with the baby's demand for food. An average infant of Sienna's age will eat one quart of formula per day. Sienna consumed two quarts per day. When Sienna was six months old, we told her mother to start feeding her solid foods. Sienna eats constantly and will scream if her mother does not feed her. She already has high cholesterol and high blood pressure.

Is Sienna obese because of her behavior? Was this learned behavior? When would she have learned this behavior, and from whom? Has she, at age one, learned to control her mother to get what she wants? Should she accept personal responsibility for her actions?

Based on "a calorie is a calorie," behaviors come first. Personal responsibility implies a choice: that there is a conscious decision leading to a behavior. This behavior is formed because of learned benefits or detriments (e.g., a child placing her hand on a stove and learning it is hot). But does this make sense with regard to obesity? In everyone? In anyone? There are six reasons to doubt "personal responsibility" as the cause of obesity.

1. Obesity Is Not a Choice

The concept of personal responsibility for obesity doesn't always make sense. In our society today, one has to ask: Are there people who see obesity as a personal advantage? Something to be desired or emulated? Across the board, modern Western societies today value the thin and shun the obese. Obesity frequently comes with many medical complications, and those afflicted are more likely to develop heart problems and type 2 diabetes (see chapter 9). Obese people spend twice as much on health care.[1] Studies show that the obese have more difficulty in dating, marriage, and fertility. The obese tend to be poorer and, even in high-paying jobs, earn less than their peers.[2]

Now ask the same question about children. Did Sienna see obesity as a personal advantage? Did she become obese on purpose? Obese children have a quality of life similar to that of children on cancer chemotherapy.[3] They are ostracized by their peers and are the targets of bullies. Many obese children suffer from low self-esteem, shame, self-hatred, and loneliness. One study showed children pictures of potential playmates. Each looked different and some had physical handicaps, such as being deformed or in a wheelchair. The researchers asked the children with whom they would rather play. The obese child came in dead last. Clearly, obesity is not something to which people, especially children, aspire.

However, this view of obesity does not necessarily square with the beliefs of obese people themselves. They see themselves as perpetrators, not victims. They often state that they know their behavior is out of control and that this behavior is their own fault. They frequently experience yo-yo dieting. They lose weight for a period of time, and when they gain it back they blame themselves, seeing the gain as a character failing. They often recount binge eating, which suggests that a degree of dietary control is lost. These experiences of losing control make them think they had the control in the first place. Did they?

2. Diet and Exercise Don't Work

If obesity were only about increased energy intake and decreased energy expenditure, then reducing intake (diet) and increasing expenditure (exercise) would be effective. If obesity were caused by learned behaviors, then changing those behaviors would be effective in reversing the process and promoting weight loss. Specific and notable successes have led to behavior/lifestyle modification as the cornerstone of therapy for obesity.

There are the anecdotal cases of weight loss by celebrities, such as Kirstie Alley or Oprah Winfrey, who publicly endorse their diets as if they were the latest fashionable handbags. They share their stories on TV and convince their viewers that this lifestyle change is possible for them, too, and that, as with adding the newest fall color to their wardrobe, losing weight will make them attractive and happy. There are reality television shows, such as *The Biggest Loser*, that document the weight loss (along with many a meltdown) of "normal people" through controlled diet and exercise. Publicity, cash prizes, and constant attention are often enough to change one's diet and exercise response for a short time. In any magazine and many infomercials, peddlers of new weight-loss remedies provide before and after pictures of people who have lost 100 pounds.

Whether this constitutes a true lasting change in behavior is doubtful. After all, Kirstie Alley and Oprah, celebrities who live in the public eye, have gained their weight back several times (until their newest miracle diet began, countless new diet books were sold, new gurus were anointed, millions of dollars were made, and the cycle repeated itself). There have been numerous reports of contestants on *The Biggest Loser* regaining much of their weight after the show ended. Most notably, Eric Chopin, the Season 3 winner, appeared on *Oprah* to tell his sorry tale of gaining at least half the weight back after his victory. He wrote in one blog post, "I'm still not back on track totally. I don't know what it is." Significant weight regain has been seen in up to one third of patients who have had surgery for weight loss (see chapter 19), because the reason for the obesity is still there. Unless it's dealt with directly, regaining will be the norm, not the exception.

Strict control of one's environment through limiting caloric intake and increasing physical activity can result in weight loss. This is true as long as the environment remains regulated. A perfect example is the army recruit who consistently loses weight due to monitored diet and vigorous exercise. This also accounts for the number of "fat schools" and "fat camps" that have sprung up nationwide. Parents send their overweight child away for the summer and are thrilled when he returns thinner, if harboring parental resentment. There are numerous reports of Hollywood stars who bulk up for a role (remember Robert DeNiro in *Raging Bull*?) and then lose the excess weight after shooting. (Of course, they have the benefit of round-the-clock personal trainers and nutritionists to monitor their food intake.) While such results are dramatic, they usually cannot be sustained. *Environmental control* is different from *behavioral control* (see chapters 17 and 18).

The real problem is not in losing the weight but in keeping it off for any meaningful length of time. Numerous sources show that almost every lifestyle intervention works for the first three to six months. But then the weight comes rolling back.[4] The number of people who can maintain any meaningful degree of weight loss is extremely small (see figure 3.1). However, because behavior/lifestyle modification is the accepted treatment, the general explanation of weight regain is that it is the individual's fault. Because he is "choosing" not to live a healthy lifestyle, the doctors and the insurance industry do not feel it their responsibility to intervene.

The same is true for children. Due to some notable and individual successes, behavior/lifestyle modification is the cornerstone of therapy. However, this is not a winning strategy for most obese children. Research shows that dietary interventions don't often work. Exercise interventions are even less successful. And unfortunately for children like Sienna, at one year of age they are unable to run on a treadmill. Also, the effects of altering lifestyle for obesity *prevention* are underwhelming and show minimal effect on behavior and essentially no effect on BMI.

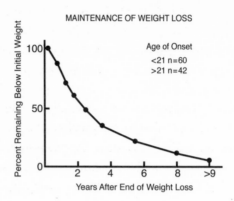

Fig. 3.1. The "Biggest Loser"—Not You. Percentage of obese individuals who were able to maintain their weight loss over nine years.

3. The Obesity Epidemic Is Now a Pandemic

If obesity were just an American phenomenon it would be an epidemic, an outbreak of illness specific to a certain area. One might then blame our American culture for promoting it. Due to our slippage in education and technological superiority, we're labeled as "fat and lazy" or "gluttons and sloths." Yet obesity is now a *pandemic*, a worldwide problem.

The United Kingdom, Australia, and Canada are right behind us. Also, in the past ten years, obese children have increased in France from 5 to 10 percent, in Japan from 6 to 12 percent, and in South Korea from 7 to 18 percent.[5] In fact, obesity and chronic metabolic diseases are occurring in underdeveloped countries that have never had such problems before.[6] Previously, poorer countries such as Malaysia had problems with malnutrition. Now Malaysia has the highest prevalence of type 2 diabetes on the planet. China has an epidemic of childhood obesity, at 8 percent in urban areas. Brazil's rate of increase in obesity is predicted to reach that of the United States by 2020. Even India, which continues to have an enormous problem with malnutrition, is not immune—since 2004, the number of overweight children increased from 17 percent to 27 percent. Sienna is not a rarity; her obese peers are being born everywhere. The areas experiencing the greatest rise in obesity and type 2 diabetes include Asia (especially the Pacific Rim) and Africa, which are not wealthy areas.[7] No corner of the globe is spared.

This is not an American problem, an Australian problem, a British problem, or a Japanese problem. This is a global problem. Could each of these countries be experiencing the same cultural shifts toward gluttony and sloth that we are? Childhood obesity knows no intellect, class, or continent.

What change in the last thirty years ties all the countries of the world together? As I mentioned in the introduction, the "American diet" has morphed into the "industrial global diet." Despite people in other countries disapproving of our fast food and TV culture, our diet has invaded virtually every other country. Our fast food culture is now global due to taste, shelf life, cost, shipping ease, and the "cool" factor (a result of effective marketing). Its acceptance is also a response to the contaminated water supplies in these areas: soft drinks are often safer, cheaper, and more available than potable water.[8] They are also cheaper and certainly more available than milk.

4. Even Animals Raised in Captivity Are Getting Fat

A recent report documented that, in the past twenty years, animals raised in captivity exhibit increasing body weights. The study examined the records of 22,000 animals of 8 different species, from rats to orangutans.[9] These animals were housed in multiple human-built colonies around the world, including labs and zoos. They don't eat our commercial food. However, their food is still processed and composed of the same general ingredients as our own. Also, these animals drink the same water and breathe the same air that we do. We don't yet know why this is happening, but the fact that even animals are showing signs of weight gain argues both against personal responsibility and in favor of some sort of environmental insult to which all life on the planet is now exposed (see chapter 15).

5. The Poor Pay More

As stated earlier, personal responsibility implies a choice, usually a conscious choice. Can one exercise personal responsibility if one doesn't have a choice? It is well known that the poor have much higher rates of obesity and chronic disease than do the rich. There are many reasons for this difference, and it is difficult to pinpoint one factor that is responsible. In the United States the poor exhibit two separate traits that argue against personal responsibility.

First, there are possible genetic issues. It is well known that African Americans and Latinos in the United States are more economically disadvantaged than their Caucasian peers. These demographic groups have higher rates of obesity than Caucasians—40 percent of Latinos and 50 percent of African Americans are obese—and are more likely to have associated medical problems, such as metabolic syndrome.[10] Certain genetic variations are more common in specific minority groups. These differences in DNA may, in part, explain the higher rates of obesity and certain metabolic diseases, such as fatty liver (see chapters 7 and 19). Genetic makeup is certainly not a choice.

Second, there are issues of access. There is a difference between the "healthy" diet of the affluent, who can purchase fresh, unprocessed foods that are high in fiber and nutrients and low in sugar, but at high prices, and, the unhealthy diet of the poor, which consists mainly of low-cost processed foods and drinks that do not need refrigeration and maintain a long shelf life. But access does not refer only to what people can afford to buy. Many poor neighborhoods throughout America lack farmers' markets, supermarkets, and grocery stores where "healthy" foods can be purchased.[11] Many supermarkets have pulled out of poor neighborhoods, mainly because of financial decisions based on revenue and fear of crime. The national supermarket chain Kroger, which is headquartered in Cincinati, in 2007 purchased twenty former Farmer Jack stores in the suburbs of Detroit, Michigan, but none within the Detroit city limits. The nearest branch is in Dearborn, eight miles away from downtown. Many who live in low-income areas also have limited access to transportation. Lower-class urban areas throughout America have been labeled "food deserts" because they are unable to sustain a healthy lifestyle. If the only place you can shop is a corner store for processed food, is what you eat really a choice? In wealthier areas of San Francisco, nearly every block has an organic food store, while in the city's poorer areas, each corner is dotted with a fast food franchise.

Even when all foods are available at low cost, the poor may not have access to refrigerators or even kitchens. Many SROs (single-room occupancy) hotels have only hot plates and no space for keeping or cooking healthy meals. Further, there is the issue of time. Many poor families are led by parents who work multiple jobs and are unable to come home and prepare healthy meals for their children, instead relying on fast food or pizza.

Lastly, the poor suffer from issues of food insecurity. People experience massive amounts of stress when they don't know where their next meal is coming from (see chapter 6). They eat what is available, when they can—usually processed food. That level of stress is incompatible with the concept of choice. Stressed people can't make a rational choice, particularly one in which short-term objectives (e.g., sating their hunger) are pitted against longer-term objectives (e.g., ensuring good health).

6. The Greatest Rate of Increase in Obesity Is in the Youngest Patients

When you look at U.S. trends in childhood obesity over the past forty years, you see that every age group is affected. However, the age group that shows the greatest rate of increase in the last decade is the two- to five-year-olds.[12] It is impossible to ascribe personal responsibility or free choice to this age group. Toddlers don't decide when, what, or how much to eat. They do not shop for or cook their own food. However, as all parents know, they do have lungs and they do make their preferences known in the supermarket. Research has shown that children are not able to tell the difference between a TV show and a commercial until they are eight years old. Children in the United States watch an average of three to four hours of TV per day. The programs are interspersed with commercials that target these young viewers and convince them of what they need.[13] If you can't discern what's marketing and what's not, how can you defend yourself against it?

We even have an epidemic of obese six-month-olds.[14] They don't diet or exercise. They drink breast milk or formula and lie in their cribs. While our society easily puts the blame on our current diet and exercise practices, how does this explain the obese six-month-old? Whatever theory you have to explain the obesity epidemic, it has to explain them also. The concept of diet and exercise in an obese infant is a non sequitur. Sienna and other obese six-month-olds lay waste to the idea of personal responsibility for obesity. Instead of perpetrator, the obese six-month-old must be a victim. But a victim of what? Or whom?

Who Is to Blame?

So we are left with a conundrum. We're all eating more and exercising less. By 2050, obesity will be the norm, not the exception. Do abnormal behaviors drive obesity? If so, behavior is primary, behavior is a choice, and personal responsibility is front and center. But what if it's the other way around? What if our biological process of weight gain drives these abnormal behaviors (see chapter 4)? To argue against personal responsibility is to argue against free will. "Free will" is defined as "the power of making free choices that are unconstrained by external circumstances or by necessity." Who is making the choices? Philosophers and scientists have argued this topic for centuries. Albert Einstein stated, "If the moon, in the act of completing its eternal way around the earth, were gifted with self-consciousness, it would feel thoroughly convinced that it was traveling its way of its own accord . . . so would a Being, endowed with higher insight and more perfect intelligence, watching man and his doings, smile about man's illusion that he was acting according to his own free will." Anthony Cashmore of the University of Pennsylvania recently proposed that free will was in reality an interaction between our DNA and our environment, along with some stochastic (random) processes.[15] Because our DNA cannot be changed, and because random processes are random, we're left with our environment, both as the sentinel exposure and the only factor than can be manipulated.

The debate about who or what is to blame for obesity will not be settled anytime soon. But I would argue that ascribing personal responsibility to the obese individual is not a rational argument for an eminently practical reason: it fails to advance any efforts to change it. The obesity pandemic is due to our altered biochemistry, which is a result of our altered environment. Part 2 will demonstrate how our behaviors are secondary, and are molded by our biochemistry.

PART II

———•———

To Eat or Not to Eat?
That's *Not* the Question

Chapter 4

Gluttony and Sloth—Behaviors Driven by Hormones

———•———

Marie is a sixteen-year-old girl with a brain tumor of the hypothalamus (the area at the base of the brain that regulates the hormones of the body). When she was ten, cranial radiation was required to kill the tumor. Since then, she has gained 30 pounds per year; she weighed 220 pounds when I first saw her. Her insulin levels spiked to incredible heights every time she ate. She had a form of intractable weight gain due to brain damage called hypothalamic obesity. She wouldn't do any activity at home, couldn't study in school, and was severely depressed. As part of a research study, I started her on a drug called octreotide, which lowered her insulin release. Within one week Marie's mother called me to say, "Dr. Lustig, something's happening. Before, we would go to Taco Bell where she would eat five tacos and an encharito and still be hungry. Now we go, she has two tacos and she's full. And she's starting to help me around the house." After beginning the medication, Marie commented to me, "This is the first time my head hasn't been in the clouds since the tumor." Within a year, she was off antidepressants and had lost 48 pounds.

Who's at fault here? Is this a case of free will? And what happened to cause Marie's reversal? If obesity is truly a result of too much energy intake (gluttony) and too little energy burned (sloth), then my last sixteen years taking care of obese children has been a complete and utter waste.

Because it's become painfully evident, after years of motivating, pleading, and arguing, that I can't change children's behavior. And I certainly can't change their parents' behavior. It was this insight from Marie, and other children like her, that exposed the inherent problems in our current thinking. Biochemistry and hormones drive our behavior.

The idea that biochemistry comes first is not a new one, but it is one that physicians, scientists, and the public should embrace. Think about the following: You see a patient who drinks ten gallons of water a day and urinates ten gallons of water a day (highly abnormal). What is wrong with him? Could he have a behavioral disorder and be a psychogenic water-drinker? Could be. Much more likely he has diabetes insipidus, a defect in a water-retaining hormone at the level of the kidney. You see a twenty-five-year-old who falls asleep in his soup. Was he up partying all night? Perhaps. But he may have narcolepsy, which is a defect in the hormone that stimulates arousal (orexins) in the midbrain. The biochemistry drives the behavior. Schizophrenia for one hundred years was a mental health disorder. Now we know that it's a defect in dopamine neurotransmission and that no amount of psychotherapy is going to help until you treat the biochemical defect. Thus, we routinely infer "biochemical" defects in many "behavioral" disturbances.

Introducing Energy Processing and Storage

To appreciate how hormones control eating behavior, first we have to look at what happens to the food we eat. In response to various brain signals (hunger, reward, stress) we ingest various calorie-laden foodstuffs (combinations of fat, protein, carbohydrate, and fiber, with some micronutrients thrown in for good measure) to build muscle and bone for growth and/or to burn for energy. These calories arrive at the stomach, a muscular bag in the abdomen about the size of a baseball glove, which releases hydrochloric acid, to begin to digest the food into smaller components. The food makes its way into the next part of the digestive tract, called the small intestine. There, a bunch of enzymes (proteins) digest the food into even smaller components, such that dietary fats are digested into fatty acids, dietary protein is sliced into amino acids, and carbohydrate is cleaved into simple sugars (mostly glucose, with varying amounts of the sweet molecule fructose). But we can't digest dietary fiber, so it remains intact. The fiber speeds the rate of transit of the food through the small intestine (see chapter 12), while limiting the rate of absorption of the other nutrients.

Once absorbed in the small intestine, the amino acids and simple sugars travel via the portal vein to the liver for immediate processing. The fatty acids are transported to the liver by a different route (the lymphatic system). The liver has first dibs on the processing of each of these three classes of nutrient. Whatever the liver can't take up appears in the general circulation. Rising levels of glucose or amino acids or fatty acids reach the pancreas, where the beta-cells release the hormone insulin.

Insulin, in common parlance, is known as the diabetes hormone. Diabetics inject insulin to lower their blood glucose. But where does the glucose go? To the fat. Insulin's actual job is to be your *energy storage hormone*. When you eat something (usually containing some form of carbohydrate), your blood glucose rises, signaling the pancreas to release insulin commensurate with the rise in blood glucose. (This is the theory behind the concept of *glycemic index*, which is discussed in chapter 17.) Insulin then tops off the liver's energy reserve by making liver starch (called glycogen), and shunts any amino acids from the blood into muscle cells. Excess fatty acids, or blood lipids, are cleared into fat cells for storage for a "rainy day," where they get turned into greasy triglycerides (such as the fat surrounding your steak). There is no energy storage without insulin—it is the key that unlocks the door to the fat cell to let energy enter and subsequently be stored as fat. Insulin makes fat—the more insulin, the more fat. And there it sits . . . and sits . . . as long as there is insulin around. When the insulin levels drop, the process goes in reverse: the triglycerides get broken down, causing the fat cells to shrink—when it happens, that's weight loss!—and the fatty acids reenter the bloodstream and travel back to the liver, where they are burned by the liver or other organs. In this way, by cycling our insulin up and down, we burn what we need, and store the rest.

Introducing the Hypothalamus

For the past sixty years we've known that the brain, especially the one cubic centimeter at the base of the brain called the hypothalamus, controls this process of energy balance. It's about the size of a thumbnail, and it is "ground zero" for the control of almost all the hormonal systems in the body.

Imagine the organization of a taxicab company. At the bottom are the taxicab drivers, getting their orders from a central dispatcher by radio and shuttling passengers all over town. The target organs—the thyroid, the adrenal, the testicles, the ovaries—are like the cabbies. They receive their orders from the central dispatcher, or, in this case, the pituitary or "master gland," which acts as the main control system. The hormones released are similar to the taxi's computerized system, signaling to the pituitary to tell it how things are going out in the field. Like the central dispatcher who directs the cabs based on their location, the pituitary will then adjust its message.

However, there is another layer of control: the chief executive officer, or CEO, who decides on hiring and firing, contracts, upgrades, and mergers and acquisitions. The company can't turn a profit without the cabbies, be efficient without the dispatcher, or be sustainable long term without a CEO. Furthermore, the CEO can alter the direction of the company based on the profitability of its cabdrivers. The CEO is akin to the hypothalamus. It sends blood-borne hormonal signals to tell the pituitary what to do. It then makes large-scale decisions based on the function of the peripheral glands, which send it information via the bloodstream. And it integrates information from other areas of the brain to alter the long-term hormonal milieu. Marie's hypothalamus was damaged beyond repair, which caused it to be ineffective in controlling her hormones and, therefore, her behavior.

The Ventromedial Hypothalamus (VMH) and Energy Balance

The hierarchy of energy balance is even more complicated. A subarea of this thumbnail is called the ventromedial hypothalamus (VMH), which serves the executive function of controlling energy storage versus expenditure. Because energy balance is *so* important to survival, there are redundant systems in case one goes amiss to ensure that the organism doesn't die.

It's clear that energy balance is the most complex function we humans perform. It's likewise apparent that energy storage, or the creation of fat cells, is the default strategy. Bottom line, we humans won't give up our hard-earned energy without a fight.

There are afferent (incoming) and efferent (outgoing) systems that control energy balance[1] (see figure 4.1). The VMH receives acute meal-to-meal information from the GI (gastro-intestinal) tract on both hunger and satiety (not shown in the figure). Either one can turn the feeling of hunger on or off by itself. But that's not all. In addition, the VMH receives more long-term information on one's fat stores and nutrient metabolism: in other words, whether your body needs to consume more calories for longer-term survival. This information is conveyed via the hormones leptin and insulin

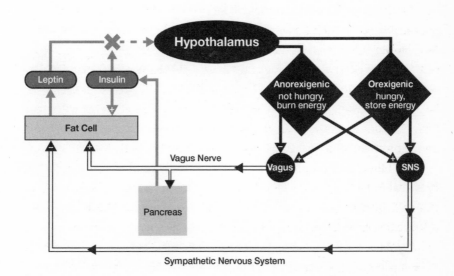

Fig. 4.1. How the Brain and Hormones Work Together (or Don't) to Regulate Energy Balance. The hypothalamus receives hormonal information from the fat cells (leptin). This information is processed into one of two signals: (a) anorexigenesis (*I'm not hungry and I can burn energy*) or (b) orexigenesis (*I'm hungry and I want to store energy*). Anorexigenesis turns *on* the sympathetic nervous system (responsible for muscle activity and fat loss), and turns *off* the vagus nerve (responsible for appetite and fat gain); while orexigenesis does the opposite. However, high insulin blocks the leptin signal, mimicking "brain starvation" and driving orexigenesis, so that we feel hungry even when we have eaten.

to the hypothalamus, where it is decoded and either stimulates or suppresses appetite, and adjusts energy expenditure accordingly.

From there, the hypothalamus sends signals from the brain to the body via two components of the autonomic nervous system. The autonomic nervous system is that portion of your body that controls your heart rate, blood pressure, and energy metabolism without your conscious effort. It is composed of two parts: the sympathetic nervous system (responsible for the fight-or-flight response) and the parasympathetic nervous system (responsible for "vegetative" functions such as food absorption and energy storage). The vagus nerve is one of the key components of the parasympathetic nervous system. There is a delicate balance and feedback loop between the sympathetic and parasympathetic systems. When that balance changes, that's when problems ensue.

The vagus nerve is fascinating. It connects the brain to all the digestive organs in the abdomen: the liver, the intestine, the pancreas, and also to the fat cells. It performs many different functions but with one ultimate goal: to store energy. The vagus is your energy storage nerve. The vagus has two parts: the afferent part (organs to brain), and the efferent part (brain to organs). The afferent vagus communicates the sensation of hunger between the stomach and brain, and also communicates information on energy processing during a meal between the liver and brain. The VMH interprets all these afferent signals, which leads to one of two physiologic states: anorexigenesis (*I don't need any more food, I can burn energy as needed, and I feel good*) or orexigenesis (*I don't have enough food, I don't want to burn any energy, and I will feel lousy until I get some more*).

The anorexigenesis signal turns on the sympathetic nervous system (SNS), which promotes energy expenditure by telling the adipose (fat) tissue and the muscles to burn energy, thereby resulting in weight loss and a sense of well-being. Anorexigenesis also turns off the vagus nerve and, in so doing, reduces appetite. Conversely, orexigenesis stimulates the vagus nerve to promote energy storage by increasing appetite. It accomplishes this by sending multiple signals through the vagus nerve: to the gastrointestinal tract to digest and absorb the food; to the adipose tissue to store more energy (make more fat); and to the pancreas to increase the amount of insulin released (promoting more energy storage into adipose tissue).

Leptin and the Elusive "Holy Grail" of Obesity

When the hormone leptin (from the Greek *Leptos*, for "thin") was discovered in 1994, for the first time, scientists thought that obesity might have a biochemical basis. Leptin has been a veritable godsend to scientists who study obesity. It provided the starting point to understanding the biochemistry of the brain pathways that control food intake and the impetus for scientists and the National Institutes of Health (NIH) to believe that there was a simple way out of this mess, one that could be easily treated with medicine and science. The U.S. government began, and continues today, to shovel money at obesity research, hoping for a treatment that works. Conversely, leptin has been the biggest disappointment to those who suffer from obesity. And woe to the pharmaceutical industry, which hoped to harness its potential for a cure and generate megabucks in the process. The pharmaceutical company Amgen was so enamored of leptin's blockbuster marketing potential that it offered $30 million for the exclusive marketing rights to the hormone, even before a human experiment had been performed. Amgen has since become so disillusioned that it has farmed leptin out to another company, Amylin Pharmaceuticals, to see if it will have better luck.

Leptin is a protein made and released by fat cells. It circulates in the bloodstream, goes to the hypothalamus, and signals the hypothalamus that you've got enough energy stored up in your fat.[2] The discovery of leptin closed the loop, providing a servomechanism (like your home's thermostat) in which the body's fat cells told the hypothalamus whether the animal was in energy surplus (obesity) or dearth (starvation). Obese animals and humans deficient in leptin respond immediately to leptin treatment with remarkable losses of fat and also with increased activity.[3] Leptin replacement corrected both behaviors, the gluttony and the sloth. The thought was, if you're obese, then your leptin doesn't work—you must be deficient and you just need more. Problem solved, right? Unfortunately, for the obese population, this simple-minded explanation was just that.

Defective Leptin Signaling: Brain Starvation

The VMH is constantly looking for the leptin signal. In the short-term, hormonal inputs can govern the size or the quality of this meal or that, but long term it's all about leptin. Leptin tells the VMH that you have enough energy on board to burn the excess, feel good, reduce your long-term food intake, and remain weight stable. When your leptin signal works, you're in energy balance, burning energy at a normal rate and feeling good.[4] Every human has a "personal leptin threshold" above which the brain interprets a state of energy sufficiency. Thus, the leptin-replete state is characterized by appropriate appetite, normal physical activity, and feelings of well-being. Woe to the 97-pound weakling who can't bulk up and gain weight; his leptin threshold is set too low, and his leptin is telling his brain to burn off any excess.

But what if leptin doesn't work or the threshold is set too high? When the VMH can't see the leptin signal, the brain interprets this as "starvation" and will direct the rest of the body to do whatever it can to increase its energy stores. The VMH relays messages to the sympathetic nervous system (SNS) to conserve energy and reduce activity. Energy expenditure is reduced by 20 percent, a great reason to feel like a sloth.[5] Furthermore, the VMH wants the body to increase energy storage. It will increase the firing of the vagus nerve in order to amplify insulin release from the pancreas and shunt more energy into fat cells, with the ultimate goal of making more leptin. The vagus makes you hungry in order that you store more energy (gluttony). Simply put, defective leptin signaling in the VMH is what brain starvation is all about. This phenomenon occurs in two ways:

Leptin deficiency. Dr. Jeff Friedman of Rockefeller University is credited with cloning the leptin gene from leptin-deficient mice,[6] which are the rodent equivalents of a 400-pound couch potato. While normal weight at birth, these mice immediately eat like there's no tomorrow and just sit there—the only time they ever get off their behinds is if you put food on the other side of the cage; then they'll waddle over to it, devour it, and sit there instead. These mice are deficient in leptin due to a genetic mutation. Their behaviors of gluttony and sloth are genetically determined. Their brain can't see their fat and in turn thinks the body is starving.

Friedman's lab also showed that giving these mice back the leptin they were missing by daily injection reduced their food intake and increased their physical activity back to normal. They lost the weight. Not only that, but all the physiological problems associated with their obesity—the diabetes, the lipid problems, and early death from heart disease—all disappeared. This made leptin look for all intents and purposes like the "holy grail" of obesity. If leptin deficiency was the cause of this pandemic, we could simply replace it, and all the unfortunate souls afflicted could be saved.

Thus far, fourteen children with mutations of the leptin gene have been identified in the entire world. These children cannot make leptin no matter how big their fat cells are, and their brains are in constant starvation mode. Amazingly, with a shot of leptin every day, they lose weight rapidly, and it's all fat (no muscle). They stop their ravenous behavior, start moving, and their puberty goes into gear.[7] For these patients, leptin is hormone-replacement therapy; while not a cure, it's the next best thing.

Leptin resistance. This is the key to the obesity epidemic. With a few rare exceptions, the other 1.5 billion overweight or obese people on the planet suffer from this. Deciphering leptin resistance is the "holy grail" of obesity. These people have plenty of leptin, and each one's blood leptin level correlates with his or her amount of body fat. This suggests that obese people are not leptin deficient but rather *leptin resistant.*[8] Their hypothalami can't see their leptin, so their brains think they're starving, and will therefore try to increase energy storage (gluttony) and conserve energy usage (sloth).

In 1999, Steven Heymsfield, then at Columbia University, gave daily injections of leptin at varying doses to obese adults for six months. All these people had high leptin levels to start. The degree of weight loss, even with the highest dosage of leptin, was underwhelming.[9] Clearly these obese people were leptin resistant. They couldn't respond to their own leptin, and no amount of extra leptin was going to make a difference. Heymsfield's study was the end of the promise of leptin as a stand-alone therapy for obesity and the end of Amgen's interest.

Hypothalamic Obesity: Behavior or Biochemistry?

This is where I enter the story. In 1995, I arrived in Memphis to start work at St. Jude Children's Research Hospital as a pediatric neuroendocrinologist. My training is in taking care of kids with brain tumors, and St. Jude had a large population of survivors. Many of these children develop hormonal deficiencies because of damage to the hypothalamus—due to the tumor itself, the neurosurgery to remove it, or the radiation and chemotherapy they receive to try to kill it. The good news is that we endocrinologists can treat these children by replacing most of the hormones that are missing—we can affect their growth, energy metabolism, and cognitive status; induce puberty when the children are age appropriate; and improve their overall health.

However, a relatively small number of children like Marie (and adults) who survive their brain tumors become *massively* obese after their tumor therapy is complete. Their hypothalamus is damaged, and their weight skyrockets. Their appetites aren't that different from those of other obese children, but their energy expenditure is markedly decreased. (Marie didn't move.) Those affected sit on the couch, watch TV, eat, poop, sleep, and generally lose interest in the world around them. As one parent stated, "It's double jeopardy. To think you might lose your kid to a cancer, and survive it, but then to lose your kid to a complication instead." Patients with this form of obesity, called hypothalamic obesity, can't lose weight. Even if these kids eat only 500 calories a day, they gain weight.[10] The neurons in the hypothalamus, which sense the leptin signal, are all dead. The "servo-mechanism" for energy balance had been short-circuited. This is leptin resistance at its worst—an *anatomic* leptin resistance. Rodent studies dating back to the early 1950s show that when you damage the VMH, the animal will become massively obese, and not even food restriction will reverse that. The VMH-lesioned rats ate more than they needed and burned less than they should have. Unlike the leptin-deficient mice, no amount of leptin would fix the problem. These animals had *anatomic* leptin resistance.[11] The leptin had no place to act.

The obese children I saw at St. Jude were similar to these VMH-lesioned rats. There was no fixing them because there was no way to regrow those neurons. Those kids were stuck forever in bodies that just kept storing energy instead of burning it,[12] with brains that constantly thought the bodies were starving. They would forever get fatter on fewer calories, never feel good, and would lose interest in everything around them. If this isn't hell on earth for parent and child, I don't know what is.

Worst yet, there was no treatment. Diet and exercise is notoriously ineffective in these children. Weight loss drugs also didn't work. In 1995, I was faced with a clinic full of patients with hypothalamic obesity following their brain tumor therapy. How to help them? I couldn't give them leptin, because the block at the hypothalamus would not allow leptin to work. If any therapy were to be successful, it would have to work downstream of the leptin neuron, somewhere between the brain and the fat cell.

Insulin: The "Leptinator"

Normally, the amount of insulin released in response to a meal is yoked to the blood sugar rise. But there are a few things that force the pancreas to make extra insulin, the vagus nerve being chief among them. When the brain can't see the leptin signal, as in children such as Marie, it interprets starvation. The vagus nerve goes into overdrive to store more energy, and kick-starts the pancreas to make extra insulin—even more than the glucose rise would predict. This excess insulin release drives nonstop energy storage and nonstop weight gain.

As it happens, there is a drug available that can lower insulin secretion as a side-effect. It is called octreotide (Sandostatin, made by Novartis Pharmaceuticals) and is what we used to treat Marie. It is normally used to reduce pituitary growth hormone secretion in patients who have tumors of the pituitary gland, a disease called acromegaly. But it also happens to reduce pancreatic insulin secretion. It doesn't wipe it out completely—that would cause diabetes—but it does reduce the rapid early release of insulin in response to a meal or a glucose tolerance test. But it's expensive, requires injections, has side-effects, and with regard to obesity, it is for experimental studies only.

We have treated many children with hypothalamic obesity with octreotide.[13] When we were successful in reducing their insulin release, the patients lost weight and started to feel better. Parents were calling me up within the first few weeks, saying, "I've got my kid back!" Most amazingly, the children had started to be active. When we got the insulin down, Marie and patients like her improved physically, mentally, and socially.

These studies highlight a crucial concept of obesity. Each of us is really two compartments: lean body mass (heart, liver, kidneys, brain, and muscles), which burns energy; and fat, which stores energy. Every molecule of energy consumed has a choice: to which compartment does the energy go? Is the energy burned or stored? Your consumption of energy is never high enough to overwhelm both compartments at the same time; no one can eat that much. This means that there is an issue of energy flux to the two compartments. What factor determines which compartment gets the energy?

Your insulin does. The more insulin there is, the more energy goes to fat. Normally your fat makes more leptin, which would feedback on your hypothalamus and decrease your insulin by reducing appetite and limiting your energy intake. In this way, the "servo-mechanism" between leptin, the brain, your pancreas, your insulin, and your fat cells maintains normal energy balance. *But* . . . if your hypothalamus can't see your leptin (in this case, because those neurons are dead from a brain tumor), then your brain thinks it's starving. It will reduce your activity to conserve energy, and increase your appetite to store more energy. When leptin doesn't work, the biochemistry comes first and the behaviors of gluttony and sloth are secondary.

This is all well and good for Marie and the few unfortunate souls with hypothalamic obesity. They have a brain tumor. They have a legitimate excuse for being fat, and at least there is now a rational, if painful and expensive, approach to treatment. For them, the biochemistry dictates the behavior. However, the overwhelming majority of obese people do not have a goombah sitting in the middle of their heads wreaking havoc on their energy balance pathway. What does this phenomenon have to do with the obesity pandemic? As you will see, everything.

Back in 1998, after three years of my working at St. Jude, the response of these patients was quite a revelation. My colleagues at the University of Tennessee and I wondered, "Is it possible that an adult population without brain tumors might manifest the same problem? Did they also have increased vagal tone driving excess insulin secretion and causing their obesity? If we gave them octreotide to suppress their insulin, might they lose weight, feel better, and start exercising?" We didn't know what these patients looked like. So we did a pilot study in forty-four morbidly obese adults recruited from off the street. We treated all of them with octreotide for six months, courtesy of Novartis Pharmaceuticals. No dieting, no exercise, just the drug. We told them, "If the drug works, it will work by itself."

We've done this experiment twice, first as a pilot and then as a placebo-controlled trial. The majority of patients did not respond to the drug. But in about 20 percent of the adults, there was big-time weight loss. The thing that predicted their success was their insulin status. The lucky responders released insulin rapidly and in high amounts at baseline, just like the brain tumor kids,[14] and their quality of life improved with the drug.

There is one final lesson to glean from these studies. All these obese adult subjects had high leptin levels. They were leptin resistant; if their leptin worked right, they wouldn't have been obese. If leptin falls, the brain should interpret this as starvation and reduce the patient's resting energy expenditure accordingly. But these patients' resting energy expenditures went up! And their improvement in energy expenditure correlated with the suppression of their insulin levels, the same as with the brain tumor kids. When we were successful in getting their insulin down, their leptin resistance improved.[15] This suggests that insulin can block leptin signaling in the brain, and therefore insulin acts as a "leptin antagonist."[16]

Many scientists have now shown that insulin actions in the VMH block leptin signaling.[17] A reduction in insulin concentrations results in a decline in leptin. Insulin and leptin are independent hormones that bind to separate receptors in the VMH. They have their own separate pathways of action, but they share the same signaling cascade. When insulin levels at the VMH are chronically high, leptin cannot signal the hypothalamus.

Deconstructing Darwin

Whenever paradoxical events occur in biology, one has to look for an evolutionary explanation. Why should insulin block leptin signaling? What's the advantage for insulin, the hormone that tells the body to store energy, to block leptin, the hormone that tells your brain to burn energy? Leptin is a necessary signal to the VMH for the initiation of high-energy processes, such as puberty and pregnancy. If leptin always worked right, then nobody could gain weight. Think of the 97-pound weakling at the beach. The crucial weight gain during puberty and pregnancy would be compromised, and our reproductive capacity would be shot. Twice in our lives we need to stop leptin from working, or we can't gain the weight, and the species dies out. Since insulin drives energy storage, it makes sense that it should do double-duty, and also be the central blocker of leptin—one hormone, two coordinated actions. Indeed, both puberty and pregnancy are hyperinsulinemic states. When adulthood or the postpartum state is reached, the insulin levels fall, weight stabilizes or is lost, and leptin levels return toward baseline.[18] However, in maladaptive conditions, when insulin is high all the time and leptin signaling is impaired, the energy gets stored yet the brain sees starvation, and obesity worsens.

When you examine the symptoms of obese and starved individuals, they are very similar. On first thought this sounds ludicrous, but it actually makes sense. Both claim fatigue, malaise, and depression. The reason for this in both groups is the inability to adequately respond to the leptin signal—in starvation because of the inadequacy of leptin, and in obesity because of the resistance to leptin. Furthermore, leptin concentrations drop precipitously during periods of short-term fasting (within twelve hours), declining faster than body fat stores. You haven't lost any weight in that time, but your fat cells are already telling your brain you're starving, driving your food intake back up. By the time you're one day into any weight-loss regimen you're already leptin deficient on top of being leptin resistant, meaning, you *really* can't see the signal. Trying not to eat for a day to fit into that little black dress? Oops. This actually drives gluttony and sloth to return your weight to its baseline level. In a nutshell, this is the recidivism of obesity. If your brain thinks there's no leptin (due to either leptin deficiency or leptin resistance) you're pretty miserable. Your sympathetic nervous system goes into conservation mode, driving down your energy expenditure, physical activity, and quality of life. Your vagus nerve then goes into overdrive, driving up your appetite, your insulin, and your energy storage.

The Alternate Interpretation of the First Law

No matter the mechanism, insulin blocks leptin signaling both in rodents and in humans. In the body, insulin causes energy storage in fat cells. In the brain, insulin causes leptin resistance and "brain starvation." Insulin delivers a one-two punch to drive gluttony and sloth, weight gain, and obesity the world over. Insulin is the bad guy in this story.

This idea turns obesity on its head. The standard thinking in obesity is: "If you eat it, you had better burn it, or you're going to store it"—in which case the weight gain is secondary to the two behaviors of increased energy intake (gluttony) and decreased energy expenditure (sloth). What these data are telling us is that it is the other way around. Storing energy is a biochemical process not under the patient's control. Burning energy is synonymous with quality of life. Things that make you burn energy faster—such as exercise, ephedrine (off the market now), and caffeine (for about two hours)—make you feel good. Conditions that make you burn energy slower—starvation and hypothyroidism, for example—make you feel lousy. So, the first law needs to be reinterpreted: "If you are going to store it, and you expect to burn it, then you will have to eat it."[19] In this interpretation, the biochemical process is primary, the weight gain is secondary, and the behaviors are a result of the biochemistry.

Obesity is a biochemical alteration in the brain promoting leptin resistance with resultant weight gain and secondary changes in behavior to maintain energy balance. The apparent character defects of gluttony and sloth are not the cause of the problem; they are the *result* of the problem. The biochemistry drives the behavior, not vice versa. The linchpin in this biochemical alteration is the hormone insulin. The majority of humans, regardless of weight, release double the insulin today that we did thirty years ago for the same amount of glucose. Now we're left with the $147 billion (the annual financial cost of obesity) question: If insulin is the bad guy and we're all hyperinsulinemic as never before in the history of humankind, where did the excess insulin come from? And how do we reverse it?

The plot thickens.   •

Chapter 5

Food Addiction—Fact or Fallacy

———————•———————

Salvador is a fifteen-year-old Latino boy with obesity, a fatty liver, and high blood pressure. He drinks four sodas a day. His mother does not buy them for him or keep them in the house. Rather, he buys them at the convenience store on the way to and from school. Salvador enrolls in our research study whereby each day, for ten days, he will consume the same number of calories from our hospital's Metabolic Kitchen, which will provide all his food, prepared by a chef and sugar free. Nonetheless, each day, he buys a can of soda and brings it home, putting it on his dresser, next to those from the day before. He tells his mother, "When the study is over, I'm drinking them all." Indeed, the evening of the end of the study, he drinks every last one, to his mother's chagrin. He may not have been addicted physically, but the mental obsession and craving indicated dependence, and could not be suppressed.

Life's too short to eat bad food, even if it's cheap. Eating is supposed to be an enjoyable experience, especially when the food is special. There's nothing quite like going to a nice restaurant with the sights, sounds, and smells of a well-prepared meal. It's one of the true enjoyments of life. Yet familiarity breeds greater cravings. Ask Philadelphians about their cheese-steaks, New Orleans denizens about their Po-Boys and beignets, or Memphians about their barbecue. Surprise! Those are among the three most obese cities in the country. Coincidence?

As prodigious as some American cuisine is, is there really anything special about a soda, a French fry, or any item in a fast food restaurant? Yet we devour fast food as if it were going out of style. Americans consume Big Macs as if each one might be our last. (Given the mortality rates in the obese, each one just might be.) Fast food comprises a growing portion of food eaten outside the home. In the United States of the 1950s, fast food accounted for 4 percent of total sales of food outside the home. In 1997 it accounted for 34 percent. Each day, 30 percent of U.S. adults eat at a fast food outlet, and McDonald's feeds forty-six million Americans.

What about the rest of the world? They didn't experience fast food growing up, yet it's now the biggest seller in developing countries. There is no familiarity here; they weren't raised on the stuff; they're consuming it *de novo*. Why do they eat fast food when it's not their traditional fare? Because it's cheap? It certainly isn't abroad. Why do the locals frequent Taco Bell in Mexico when the original tacos are cheaper and ostensibly healthier? Something more is going on here. Is the world addicted to fast food? The biology of addiction is at the center of this question.

Might as Well Face It, We're Addicted to . . .

Our brains are wired for reward—it is the primary force behind human survival. Reward is the reason to get up in the morning. If you take away reward, you take away the reason to live. We know this from recent experience with the anti-obesity drug rimonabant, which was deep-sixed after it failed to gain approval from the FDA in 2007. Rimonabant is an endocannabinoid antagonist, or the "anti-marijuana" medicine—which means it's also "anti-munchies." It inhibits the sense of reward. While it worked to promote weight loss, 20 percent of the subjects who used it experienced serious psychiatric side effects, especially depression, and there were several suicides. Kill the reward system, and you just might want to kill yourself.

Although the brain's reward system is complex and has many inputs, it can be reduced to the "hedonic pathway." This pathway is where primal emotions, reproductive drive, and the survival instinct are all housed and expressed. These reward mechanisms are thought to have evolved to reinforce behaviors that are essential for perpetuation of the species and survival: such as sex for reproduction and the enjoyment of food so that you eat. This is also the pathway that reinforces the positive and negative aspects of drugs of abuse such as nicotine, cocaine, morphine, and alcohol. In order to maintain eating as one of the most powerful urges in animal and human behavior, evolution has also made it a rich source of pleasure and reward.

The hedonic pathway comprises a neural conduit between two brain areas: the ventral tegmental area (VTA) and the nucleus accumbens (NA, also known as the reward center), both of which are deep-brain structures. Pleasure occurs when the VTA signals the NA to release dopamine, a neurotransmitter. It's a signal from one brain center to another. When the released dopamine binds to its specific dopamine D_2 receptor in the NA, the sense of pleasure is experienced.[1]

So what are neurotransmitters and receptors? Think of keys and locks. Each neuron is a cell body, and at its end is an axon (special fiber of the neuron that sends information). This axon has a synapse, or pathway, that connects to the dendrites (specialized fibers of the nerve cell that receive information) of the next neuron. When a neural impulse is generated in the first cell, it pulses down to the end of the axon, which contains little packets of neurotransmitters that are then released. These are the keys. They travel across the synapse to the receptors (locks), located in the dendrites of the next cell. There are many keys that take the path along the synapse, and not all of them make it to their destination. Along their way via the synapse, some are metabolized and some are "re-uptaken." Dopamine is one of these types of keys traveling to fit into the locks of the D_2 receptors in the next cell, thus determining the triggering and firing of the next cells down the chain.

Food intake is just one readout of the hedonic pathway.[2] It appears to mediate feeding on the basis of palatability rather than energy need: *I'm stuffed, but that chocolate cake looks so good.* When functional, the hedonic pathway helps to curtail food intake in situations where energy stores are replete: *I don't need to finish that macaroni and cheese.* However, when dysfunctional, this pathway can increase food intake, leading to obesity.

If you feed a rodent a palatable food (e.g., a high-fat, high-sugar food such as cookie dough), the animal experiences reward because dopamine is released from the VTA and binds to the D_2 receptor in the NA. As long as that continues, the animal will continue to eat and experience reward. There are three processes that modulate this system in one direction or another:

1. Anything that increases the dopamine transmission to the NA increases the feeling of reward.
2. Anything that clears dopamine from the NA will extinguish the feeling of reward.
3. Anything that reduces the number of D_2 receptors in the NA, or binding of dopamine to those receptors (such as chronic overuse of a substance), will shortchange reward. You then need more dopamine, and hence more of the substance, to get the same feeling of pleasure.

These precepts are as true for food as they are for addictive drugs. And food and drugs cross over. With time we can become sensitized to a substance and need more of it to get the same effect. Once sensitized, animals and humans may become hyperresponsive to a new substance; this is known as cross-sensitization. In other words, if the brain has been wired for addiction, it's easy to switch from one substance to another. Ask recovering alcoholics about their incessant need for coffee, tobacco, and/or sugar. A reinforcer is a stimulus that increases the probability that an animal or human will respond to the addictive drug. Food is a form of positive reinforcement. Dopamine stimulation in the NA reinforces the intake of drugs or alcohol and also of food.

The reinforcing effect of dopamine is attributed to D_2 receptor stimulation. As stated before, food intake increases as a result of morphine and marijuana use. The film *Harold and Kumar Go to White Castle* details the odyssey of two very stoned guys who seek to overcome seemingly insurmountable obstacles in their quest for a hamburger. We can measure this by dopamine release and D_2 receptor signaling. Why does dopamine matter so much? In a normal person, dopamine will be cleared from the D_2 receptors after he is satiated. If you have a decreased dopamine binding capacity, there is a perceived need for compulsive food intake to provide excess stimulation of these depressed circuits, thereby driving continued weight gain.

The Usual Suspects: Leptin and Insulin

Yup, them again. Not only are they central in the starvation response, but they are also key players in this hedonic pathway, modulating reward in response to meals. In normal circumstances, after you've eaten a sufficient amount, leptin sends a signal to the VTA to suppress the release of dopamine, thereby reducing the reward of food.[3]

So leptin extinguishes reward. But what if you are leptin resistant? That's what obesity is: leptin resistance. If leptin can't act, then the dopamine isn't cleared from the NA, and the impetus for further consumption persists. If you're leptin resistant, do you really think you have the willpower to ignore both the starvation signal *and* the reward signal, when every food outlet you pass by provides you with sight or smell cues to chow down? Starvation and reward conspire to thwart every obese person.

What about insulin, leptin's accomplice? Normally, people are sufficiently sensitive to insulin. Insulin's job is to clear dopamine from the synapses (that pathway between the cells) in the NA.[4] Thus, the rise in insulin that occurs during a meal blunts the reward of further food intake (*I've eaten enough—I really don't need a second helping*). This acts as a servomechanism built into the hedonic pathway to prevent overfeeding. But what happens when you are insulin resistant? Insulin resistance leads to leptin resistance in the VTA, contributing to increased caloric intake by preventing dopamine clearance from the NA. Increased pleasure is then derived from food when energy stores are full.[5] Insulin and leptin resistance lead not only to increased food intake but to increased *palatable* food intake or anything that is high in both fat and sugar: the muffins, the Cinnabons, the cookies, the cheesecake. Is it any wonder Mrs. Fields is in every shopping mall?

Defining Food Addiction: Liking, Wanting, and Needing

Look, we all like fast food. And why wouldn't we? It's designed to contain the greatest concentration of fat, sugar, salt, and caffeine, and is placed into as small a package as possible. Yummmm. It provides food cheaply, quickly, and without table service. The pretty packaging and restaurant environment increase its salience (the properties that make you like it more). Ten years ago, fast food locations in the United States generated more than $125 billion, which accounts for 15 percent of sales of the *entire* U.S. food industry. But *liking* it isn't the same as *wanting* it. And *wanting* it isn't the same as *needing* it.[6]

Liking is an aesthetic state. You can turn it on and turn it off. As dopamine is released into the NA, our consumption of a Big Mac heightens our sense of reward. Then comes the insulin rush, and that should be the end of it. But when you're insulin resistant, *wanting* is a psychological state and *needing* becomes a physiologic state. You can't turn it on and off anymore. This is the nature of addiction to any substance of abuse. It's what happens with nicotine, morphine, cocaine, and alcohol—and it happens with food. It can happen to anyone. It can happen to you.

Substance dependence, in this case synonymous with addiction, is defined by the American Psychological Association (APA) as "a maladaptive pattern of substance abuse leading to clinically significant impairment or distress." There is currently no standardized definition for food addiction despite many hypotheses in the medical literature. There are seven criteria for substance dependence according to the APA *Diagnostic and Statistical Manual*, the DSM-IV-TR. The first two are considered physiologic, whereas criteria 3–7 are considered psychological dependence. All these are seen in the obese, especially those who frequent fast food restaurants. To be considered addicted to any substance of abuse, one must meet at least three of the seven.

1. **Tolerance.** This is defined as the need for more substance to get the same effect, or when the same amount of substance produces less effect with continued use. That Big Mac still generates the dopamine rush, but the reward isn't maintained, as your insulin won't clear the dopamine from the NA. Since insulin resistance generates leptin resistance, you can't stop the dopamine neurons in the VTA from firing in the first place. So your NA is awash in dopamine, and the insulin rush from the meal can't turn it off. Since your hypothalamus *and* your NA won't respond to the leptin signal, the drive to eat just keeps coming. And here's the kicker: the more and the longer your NA is exposed to dopamine, the more those D_2 receptors are going to be down-regulated. After chronic dopamine exposure, the D_2 receptors themselves start to disappear. The locks vanish, much to the chagrin of the keys, which have nowhere to go. Now it takes more dopamine to ensure that the few receptors that don't disappear are occupied. You need to eat more Big Macs just to get the same level of reward.

2. **Withdrawal.** This is characterized by physical signs (such as tremors) and psychological ones (anxiety, depression). This occurs due to lack of dopamine D_2 receptor occupancy. In animals, anxiety and depression are indicated by unwillingness to spend time in a risky environment. In humans, withdrawal is expressed as symptoms of depression and anxiety. If you try to stop eating those Big Macs, your dopamine drops and you are consumed by feelings of anxiety and depression (just like those patients treated with rimonabant—the "anti-munchie" medicine). The only choice is to increase the dopamine, reoccupy those diminished D_2 receptors, and maintain the vicious cycle of Big Mac consumption.

If you need proof, I suggest you rent the 2004 documentary *Super Size Me.* The film's author and star, Morgan Spurlock, began as a reasonably healthy specimen at 6 feet 2 inches and 185 pounds (for a BMI of 23.8, within the normal range). He was eating a reasonably healthy diet (his girlfriend was a vegan chef) before beginning a thirty-day ordeal of eating every meal at McDonald's. By day eighteen, he relates to the camera, "You know, I was feeling awful. I was feeling like s--t. I was feeling sick, and un-happy. . . . Started eating; now I feel great. I feel so great, it's crazy." Mr. Spurlock just described withdrawal. In eighteen days, he went from being a person with healthy eating habits to a fast food addict.

3. **Bingeing.** This is defined as an escalation of intake, using a greater amount of the substance or using for a longer duration than intended. In animals, this can be measured by an increase in the number of times the animal presses a lever to self-administer a drug—or, in the case of a human, continuing to eat after satiety has been achieved. One can easily conceptualize binge drinking (think of the movie *Animal House* or your stereotypical chug-a-lug frat guy), but binge eating is harder to define. It is highly subjective, since what is a large amount to some may not be perceived as unusual by others. Binge eating disorder includes eating until uncomfortable; eating when not hungry; eating alone due to shame; feeling disgusted, depressed, or guilty after overeating; and marked distress over the bingeing. Many afflicted people will consume massive amounts of food, such as an entire sheet cake, alone and in the dark of their kitchen, with massive shame.

4. **Desire or attempts to cut down or quit.** As mentioned previously, diets and miracle drugs generate over $160 billion annually. Those who are overweight or obese are almost always on some new diet kick and are frequently "weight cycling," or yo-yoing. Juicing, cleansing, meat only, carbs only—they grasp for any possible solution. And it's almost never sustainable. After a period of days, weeks, or months, they frequently binge on the substance from which they were abstaining (often sugar), and the weight is gained back. The sense of failure and ensuing depression can be overwhelming. The obese then read a new article or book about the latest craze and begin the cycle again *ad infinitum*. It's not that they aren't trying. Their lives are often consumed by these attempts.

5. **Craving or seeking.** This is described as an intense drive to self-administer drugs. In food addiction research, craving is illustrated by the motivation to seek food. Drug craving and seeking have been experimentally described as a form of learning, where dopamine signaling facilitates the consolidation of memory; past experiences are used to inform future

decisions. Rats "press the lever" for drugs because they have learned that it is rewarding. We press the credit card button for Frappucinos™.

6. **Interference with life.** This is defined by important work, social, or other life activities being compromised. Obesity can significantly hamper an individual's quality of life. Mobility is markedly more difficult. Airlines may refuse you passage if you don't fit into the seat. Employers may refuse to hire you based on your weight. Diabetes can lead to limb amputation, requiring use of a wheelchair. During the thirty days of Spurlock's *Super Size Me* adventure, he gained 24.5 pounds, experienced mood swings, sexual dysfunction, and fat accumulation in his liver. While his experience of eating every meal at McDonald's may be deemed extreme, these physical and physiological effects occurred within only a thirty-day period.

7. **Use despite negative consequences.** This is defined as continued use despite knowledge that use will make the problems worse. The health consequences associated with obesity are numerous (see chapter 19). Despite knowing and experiencing these health problems, the eating pattern continues unabated.

What Makes Fast Food Addictive?

In humans, food addiction is often compared to established criteria for substance dependence.[7] One problem with this approach is that it shifts focus away from the potentially addictive properties of the food and onto the individual "afflicted" with the addiction. We prefer to focus on the addictive potential of the food itself by placing it in the scope of other identified substances of abuse. Alcohol is the most analogous substance to fast food for several reasons, including its biochemistry (see chapters 11 and 22).

Fast food is high in calories, sugar, fat, salt, and caffeine. It is highly processed, energy dense, and specifically designed to be highly palatable. The majority of the fiber and a portion of the vitamins and minerals present in the original food have been extracted in processing (see chapter 14). Sugar, salt, and other additives are used to boost flavor. The end product is packaged and sold conveniently to deliver the contents. Which of these components could be addictive? Or are they addictive all together?

A market share analysis of McDonald's, the largest hamburger chain in the world, shows that its Big Mac and French fries are the top two most popular menu items. Extra value meals constitute 70 percent of purchases at McDonald's, Wendy's, and Burger King. The most popular combination at McDonald's is a Big Mac, medium French fries, and medium regular soda, providing 1,130 calories for $5.99.[8]

But we're talking about addiction here. So let's make it a large. Consider a food label for a typical fast food meal, consisting of a Big Mac, large French fries, and large Coke (32 ounces) (figure 5.1). No percentage daily value (%DV) is listed for sugar because there is currently no recommended daily intake for

Nutrition Facts

Serving Size 1 Big Mac, 1 large French fries, 1 Large Coke (1,269g)

Amount Per Serving

Calories 1,360	Calories from Fat 520

% Daily Value*

Total Fat 58g	**89%**
Saturated Fat 12g	**58%**
*Trans*Fat 1.5g	
Cholesterol 80g	**89%**
Sodium 80g	
Total Carbohydrate 190g	**63%**
Dietary Fiber 10g	**40%**
Sugars 95g	
Protien 32g	

Vitamin A 8%	•	Vitamin C 20%
Calcium 30 %	•	Iron 30%

* Percent Daily Values are based on a 2,000 calorie diet. You Daily Values may be higher or lower depending on your calorie needs:

	Calories:	2,000	2,500
Total Fat	Less than	65g	80g
Sat Fat	Less than	20g	25g
Cholesterol	Less than	300mg	300mg
Sodium	Less than	2,400mg	2,400mg
Total Carb		300g	375g
Dietary Fiber		25g	30g

Fig. 5.1. Supersize Me? A McDonald's Meal and Its Nutritional Value. A Big Mac, large fries, and a large soda provide 1,360 calories (two thirds of a standard day's allotment) and 1,380 milligrams sodium (almost an entire day's allotment). While the fat content is 38 percent of calories (which is not bad), the sugar content is 95 grams, or 19 teaspoons, or 390 calories, which is more than double what the American Heart Association recommends for one day.

sugar (see chapter 16). Keep in mind that 50 percent of the American population is consuming this or a similar meal at least once per week.

Salt

This sample meal contains 1,380 milligrams of sodium (salt). The 2005 Dietary Guidelines for Americans provided a "tolerable upper intake level" of 2,300 milligrams of sodium per day, which is why the %DV of the sample meal is 54 percent. Processed foods of many sorts contribute more than 3,400 milligrams of sodium per day to the average American diet. Salt is one method by which the food industry can preserve foods and increase their shelf life. So salt and calories almost always go together. (Think potato chips.) But is it addictive? Data to support addiction to salt are currently confined to animal models. Studies in rats show dopamine signaling in response to salt, and administration of opioids encourages bingeing on salt. However, in humans, salt intake has traditionally been conceived as a learned preference rather than an addiction. The preference for salty foods is likely learned early in life. Four- to six-month-old infants establish a salt preference based on the sodium content of breast milk, water used to mix formula, and the rest of their diet. But clearly people can modulate their salt intake. For example, patients who crave salt due to diseases of the adrenal gland can reduce their salt intake when given the appropriate medicine. Also, people's taste for salt can be retrained; hypertensive adults can be retrained to a lower-salt diet within twelve weeks.[9] So, based on the criteria for an addictive substance, salt doesn't make the cut.

Fat

The high fat content of fast food is vital to its rewarding properties. This sample fast food meal contains 89 percent of the daily fat intake for an individual on a 2,000-calorie diet. In feeding studies, excess calories from fat are more efficiently stored than excess calories from carbohydrates (90–95 percent versus 75–85 percent). Therefore, fat intake has always traditionally been assumed to be the major determinant of weight gain. Animals will binge on pure fat when given intermittent access to it. They binge regardless of the type of fat ingested, which suggests that it is that fat *content* and not the type of fat present in fast food that encourages overeating (see chapter 10). However, rat models do not demonstrate other features of addiction to fat, such as tolerance or withdrawal. Keep in mind, however, that so-called "high-fat foods" are almost always also high in starch (e.g., pizza) or sugar (e.g., cookies). In fact, adding sugar significantly enhances preference for high-fat foods among normal-weight people.[10] Thus, the combination of high fat along with high sugar is likely to be more addictive than high fat alone.

Caffeine

Soda is an integral part of the fast food meal. If you consumed a large soda with your McDonald's value meal, the caffeine content would be approximately 58 milligrams. Soft drink manufacturers identify caffeine as a flavoring agent in their beverages, but only 8 percent of frequent soda drinkers can detect the difference in a blind taste test of caffeine-containing and caffeine-free cola.[11] Thus, the most likely function of the caffeine in soda is to increase the salience (the quality that makes it "stand out") of an already highly rewarding (sugared) beverage. Dependence on caffeine is well established, meeting all the DSM-IV-TR criteria for both physiologic and psychological dependence. In fact, up to 30 percent of people who consume caffeine may meet the criteria for dependence. Headache (attributed to increased cerebral blood flow velocity), fatigue, and impaired task performance have all been shown during caffeine withdrawal. In addition, reinforcement of intermittent caffeine consumption leads to tolerance.

While children get their caffeine from soft drinks and chocolate, adults get most of their caffeine from coffee and tea. An 8-ounce cup of brewed coffee contains 95–200 milligrams of caffeine, depending on how it is brewed. The late comedian and social commentator George Carlin famously referred to coffee as "Caucasian crack." However, few customers these days order a regular brewed coffee at chain restaurants. A study of Starbucks customers showed that the majority of them order blended drinks.[12] The ever popular "grande" (extra large) Mocha Frappuccino (without whipped cream) has 260 calories and 53 grams of sugar. Thus, as a known substance of abuse, caffeine in coffee drinks and soda is part and parcel of the phenomenon of food addiction.

Sugar

Although anecdotal reports abound supporting human "sugar addiction," we are still not completely sure whether this is full-fledged dependence or merely habituation. Adding a soda to a fast food meal increases the sugar content tenfold. While Coca-Cola estimates that currently 42 percent of soft drinks sold nationwide are diet drinks (e.g., Coke Zero), when purchased at McDonald's, 71 percent are the sugar-sweetened variety. In fact, in 2009 only seven items on the McDonald's menu did not include sugar—French fries, hash browns, sausage, Chicken McNuggets (without dipping sauce), Diet Coke, black coffee, and iced tea (without sugar). While soda intake is independently related to obesity,[13] fast food eaters clearly drink more soda. It is likely that the widespread phenomenon of "soda addiction" is driven by the inclusion of caffeine, a known addictive substance.

All criteria for sugar addiction have been demonstrated in rodent models.[14] First, rats exposed to intermittent sugar access (following restriction) will binge. Second, these animals show signs of withdrawal (teeth chattering, tremors, shakes, and anxiety) when the sugar is withdrawn. Third, seeking and craving have been demonstrated where animals consume more sugar after a two-week imposed abstinence—just like Salvador and his soda. Elevated dopamine levels perpetuate the binge, and overconsumption increases with time, consistent with tolerance. Finally, cross-sensitization has been demonstrated in sugar-addicted rats who readily switch to alcohol or amphetamine use. So, based on the data, sugar is addictive, and soda is doubly so.

Deconstructing Darwin

There is some evidence that sugar may be addictive in humans. Experimental studies show that obese subjects will use sugar to treat psychological symptoms. Overweight women who were self-reported carbohydrate cravers reported greater relief from various mood disorders in response to a carbohydrate-containing beverage as compared to a protein drink. But perhaps the best evidence for an opiate-like effect of sugar is the product Sweet-Ease. This is a sugar solution into which hospitals dip pacifiers for newborn boys undergoing circumcision, to reduce the pain of the procedure.

Evolutionarily, sweetness was the signal to our ancestors that something was safe to eat because no sweet foods are acutely poisonous. (Even Jamaican vomiting sickness occurs only after consumption of unripe ackee fruit, which is not sweet.) So we gravitate to sweetness as a default. How many times do parents have to introduce a new food before a baby will accept it? About ten to thirteen times. But if that new food is sweet, how many times do you have to introduce it? Only once. And if a sucrose solution on a pacifier can provide enough analgesia for performing a circumcision, that's an evolutionary winner, isn't it?

Pleasure versus Happiness

You may have heard of the "gross national happiness index," an indicator that measures quality of life or social progress in more psychological terms than does the economic indicator of gross domestic product (GDP). By all accounts, America is not very happy. Despite having the highest GDP, we score forty-fourth on the happiness index. Of course, our workaholic attitudes (Americans are afforded the least vacation time in the developed world) and the recent economic downturn all contribute to our unhappiness. But could our unhappiness be related to our food?[15]

By all estimations, obese people are not happy. The question is whether their unhappiness is a cause or a result of their obesity. At this point we can't say for sure, and it is entirely possible that both are correct. Here's how.

Happiness is not just an aesthetic state. Happiness is also a biochemical state, mediated by the neurotransmitter serotonin. The "serotonin hypothesis" argues that deficiency of brain serotonin causes severe clinical depression, which is why selective serotonin reuptake inhibitors (SSRIs) which increase brain serotonin, such as Wellbutrin and Prozac, are used as treatment. Interestingly, these medications are also used for obesity. One way to increase serotonin synthesis in the brain is to eat lots of carbohydrates.[16]

You can see where this is going. If you're serotonin-deficient, you're going to want to boost your serotonin any way you can. Eating more carbohydrates, especially sugar, initially does double duty: it facilitates serotonin transport and it substitutes pleasure for happiness in the short term. But as the D_2 receptor down-regulates, more sugar is needed for the same effect. The insulin resistance drives leptin resistance (see chapter 4), and the brain thinks it's starved, driving a vicious cycle of consumption to generate a meager pleasure in the face of persistent unhappiness. And this vicious cycle can happen to anyone. Just substitute a little pleasure for a little unhappiness, and presto! Addiction in no time at all.

You, the Jury . . .

There is one obvious hole in this thesis, and I'm sure you've been chomping on it throughout this entire chapter. Can anyone become addicted to fast food? Everyone in America eats fast food, but not everyone is addicted. With narcotics, chronic use pretty much assures addiction—ask Rush Limbaugh about his OxyContin—but fast food doesn't fit this paradigm. There are lots of habitual fast food consumers who can stop if they wished. Instead, is there a subset of people who are "addictable" and who have chosen food as their preferred substance of abuse? This might explain why people who stop smoking start eating.

Doctors are starting to come around to the concept of food addiction. Nora Volkow, the head of the National Institute on Drug Abuse (NIDA) is on record supporting the concept of food addiction.[17] Yet not everyone is sold on the idea that obesity and addiction are related. For instance, in 2012 a British group challenged the obesity-addiction model,[18] arguing that not

all obese people demonstrate addiction, that not all obese people have reduced dopamine receptors on neuroimaging, and that rats are not humans
(although, of course, some humans are rats). By that token, not everyone
who drinks becomes an alcoholic, but we do know that some people become addicted.

So what's your verdict? Is Salvador addicted to his sodas? Is fast food
addictive? After treating obese children for the last fifteen years, I can cat-
egorically say that there are loads of people who can't kick the habit. In fact,
it's more likely that children are unable to—perhaps because they were
raised on the stuff or because their brains are more susceptible.[19] There are
several caveats to declaring fast food addictive. How often do you partake
(consistently or intermittently)? With whom do you partake (with your
family, or alone)? What do you order? How old are you? And, most important, do you have a soda (or sweet tea in the southeastern United States)
with your meal? I've laid out the data that demonstrate that fat and salt increase the appeal of the fast food meal, but it's the sugar and the caffeine
that are the true hooks. We'll come back to this time and again throughout
the book, as this is where the action is.

Chapter 6

Stress and "Comfort Food"

———————●———————

Janie is thirteen years old. When she was five she developed a hypothalamic brain tumor, which was surgically removed. In the subsequent seven years, she gained 160 pounds (to a maximum weight of 242 pounds) and her oral glucose tolerance test showed massive insulin release, consistent with hypothalamic obesity. On an experimental protocol, our surgeons performed an experimental operation on Janie, which cut her vagus nerve. In the nine months following the surgery, she lost 22 pounds, reduced her hunger, had more energy, and felt much better. Then she disappeared from the clinic for nine months. When she returned, she had regained the 22 pounds and was back up to her maximum weight. She stated that the surgery had removed her hunger. So how and why did she gain it all back? It turns out she switched schools in sixth grade. The kids in the new school hurled insults, calling her Fatso, Miss Piggy, and The Blob. Despite a lack of hunger, the stress of her new situation caused her to eat incessantly. Janie switched to a new middle school, where she got along better with her peers, and lost weight again.

This poor young lady is triply cursed. First she gets a brain tumor. Then she gets obese as a complication of the brain tumor. To top it all off, she has the misfortune of being a teenager (possibly the worst of the three). Even though we did our best to treat this girl's biochemical difficulty, the social difficulty turned out to be even more potent.

I take care of kids for a living. While the majority of them are cute and adorable, some kids can be downright mean. Especially adolescents. Bad behavior is *de rigueur* nowadays. How many movies out of Hollywood play on this adage? Rent *Mean Girls, Sixteen Candles*, or *Can't Buy Me Love* in case you've forgotten what high school is like. Maybe it's the testosterone and estrogen of puberty that makes some teenagers angry and turns them into bullies. Perhaps they build themselves up by taking other kids down with degrading remarks and slurs. Maybe it's their upbringing. They see how their parents handle social issues and they emulate them. (Beware the mothers of the PTA in the San Fernando Valley.) But I do know one thing: many kids (and adults) respond to psychological stress by eating.

Coincident with the rise in obesity throughout our society is an increased prevalence and severity of psychological stress.[1] Two mechanisms by which stress leads to obesity are stress-induced eating and stress-induced fat deposition.[2] Both animals and humans have been documented to increase their food intake following stress or negative emotion, even if the organism is not hungry. Further, the type of food eaten tends to be high in sugar, fat, or both. There's a load of evidence that humans are more stressed today than we were thirty years ago, which correlates directly with the expansion of our waistlines.

Cortisol: Can't Live with It, Can't Live Without It

The relationship between stress, obesity, and metabolic disease begins with the hormone cortisol, which is released by your adrenal glands (located on top of your kidneys). This is perhaps the most important hormone in your body. Too little cortisol, and you can die. If you're missing any other hormone in your body—growth, thyroid, sex, or water-retaining hormones—you'll feel lousy and your life will be miserable, but you won't perish. But if you're missing cortisol, you can't handle any form of physical stress. As David Williams stated in the 2008 PBS series *Unnatural Causes*, "Stress helps to motivate us. In our society today everybody experiences stress. The person who has no stress is a person who is dead." The acute rise in cortisol keeps you from going into shock when you dehydrate, improves memory and immune function, reduces inflammation, and increases vigilance. Normally cortisol will peak in a stressful situation (when you're being chased by a lion or your boss is yelling at you for not getting the memo). Cortisol is necessary, in small doses and in short bursts.

Conversely, long-term exposure to large doses of cortisol will also kill you—it'll just take longer. If pressures (social, familial, cultural, etc.) are relentless, the stress responses remain activated for months or even years. When cortisol floods the bloodstream, it raises blood pressure; increases the blood glucose level, which can precipitate diabetes; and increases the heart rate. Human research shows that cortisol specifically increases caloric intake of "comfort foods" (e.g., chocolate cake).[3] And cortisol doesn't cause just any old weight gain. It specifically increases the visceral fat (see chapter 8), which is the fat depot associated with cardiovascular disease and metabolic syndrome.

Beginning in the 1970s and lasting more than thirty years, the seminal "Whitehall study" charted the health of twenty-nine thousand British civil servants.[4] In the beginning, the scientists hypothesized that the high-power executives would have the highest rates of heart attack and coronary disease. The opposite proved to be true. Those lowest on the totem pole exhibited the highest levels of cortisol and of chronic disease. This held true not just on the bottom rung: the second person down on the social ladder had a higher likelihood of developing diseases than the person on the top rung, the third had a higher predisposition than the second, and so on. Death rates and illness correlate with low social status, even after controlling for behavior (e.g., smoking).

The same holds true in America. The prevalence of diseases such as diabetes, stroke, and heart disease are highest among those who suffer from the most stress, namely middle- and lower-class Americans. These stressors are acutely felt in children as well. Almost 20 percent of American children live in poverty. The lifelong consequences of food and housing insecurity are toxic to the brain and alter its architecture early in life.[5] In particular, cortisol kills neurons that play a role in the inhibition of food intake.[6] Whether one builds a strong or weak foundation in childhood is a great determinant of later health and eating patterns. Thus, childhood stress increases the risk of obesity during adolescence and adulthood.

Some of the factors associated with lower thresholds for stress and higher "cortisol reactivity" are low socioeconomic status, job stress, being female, scoring high in dietary restraint (a measure of chronic dieting), and an overall lack of power and confidence. Taking three buses to get anywhere, working two or more jobs, figuring out how to put food on the table, and not knowing whether you will be able to pay the rent—all significantly affect not just your state of mind but also your physiological state. And if you are not Caucasian, the stresses associated with racism will double these health effects. African Americans and Latinos suffer from higher mortality rates of nearly every disease than their white counterparts. While there are certainly genetic influences, stress plays a major role in health disparities among the races.

The Science of Stress

The stress response is a cascade of adaptive responses that originate in the central nervous system. When an individual perceives stress (anything from a plane crash to a calculus test), the body interprets and processes the threat in an area of the brain called the amygdala. From there, the amygdala switches on two other systems. First, like a game of telephone, the amygdala tells the hypothalamus, which tells the pituitary, which tells the adrenal gland to release cortisol. In an acute situation, cortisol feeds back on the hypothalamus to stop further secretion, and its effects would be short term and limited. (*I escaped the lion! Ah, sweet relief. Time for a nap.*) This negative feedback loop should protect the brain and body from prolonged, detrimental cortisol exposure. Second, the amygdala activates the sympathetic nervous system (SNS), raising the heart rate. Both cortisol and the SNS raise blood sugar and blood pressure, to prepare the individual for meeting and adapting to stress. These systems should shut off after the stress has passed.

However, either chronic stress or heightened responses to stress due to ineffective coping strategies will unleash a long-term cortisol cascade. In these prolonged stressful situations, the cortisol is unregulated. Why doesn't the cortisol feed back in the state of chronic stress to control its own release? This is one of the biggest questions in science today. Apparently, the amygdala's ability to perceive the cortisol signal becomes reduced in response to the excess cortisol supply. Chronic exposure suppresses the negative feedback of cortisol on the brain. How and why this happens is still unknown. Whatever the mechanism, it's a vicious cycle: stress breeds more cortisol, which in turn breeds more stress.[7]

"Stressed" Is "Desserts" Spelled Backward

Over several years, prolonged cortisol leads to excessive food intake—but not just *any* food. Human research shows that cortisol specifically increases caloric intake of "comfort foods" (those with high energy density or high fat and high sugar). Your spouse is late and the kids won't stop whining? Break out the Ben & Jerry's.

What predisposes certain people to stress-induced eating? For one thing, it's not the stress itself; it's the *response* to stress. Stress, like art, is in the eye of the beholder. The same level of stress can have varying effects on different people. The perception of chronic stress causes increased caloric intake of "comfort foods," but only among those with high cortisol reactivity. People who are "stress eaters" exhibit significant increases in insulin, weight, and cortisol at night (normally the time for cortisol to be very low) during a stressful period. My colleague Elissa Epel at the University of California, San Francisco showed that those subjects who generated the greatest amount of cortisol in response to a psychological stressor also consumed the greatest amount of high-fat, sugary food.[8] Stress has also been postulated to play a role in metabolic syndrome in childhood, a time when eating patterns and fat cells are "programmed."

Stress may affect food intake in several ways. One outcome of stress is reduced sleep, which is both a contributor to and a consequence of obesity. We're all getting less sleep than we used to, especially children (Janie included).[9] BMI increases over time among short sleepers. And just because you sleep less does not mean you are filling your waking hours with exercise. At the biochemical level, acute sleep loss is associated with elevations in markers of systemic inflammation and signs of metabolic syndrome.

Sleep deprivation has been shown to increase cortisol and reduce leptin, and in doing so, mimic starvation and hunger. At the brain level, sleep deprivation increases the hunger hormone ghrelin, which increases the "value" each of us puts on food, and also activates the reward system,[10] making you eat even more chocolate cake. Conversely, poor sleep is common among obese individuals. This is in part because high BMI is a strong predictor of obstructive sleep apnea, which, due to retention of carbon dioxide, appears to make obesity even worse.

The role of stress and cortisol in eating extends from the physiologic to the pathologic, and from overeating to undereating. When I was a pediatric resident working thirty-six hours out of every forty-eight, our group was divided into two cohorts: those who hit the cafeteria and those who lived on coffee. I tried the coffee, but my hands shook too much when I was threading catheters into umbilical arteries on premature infants, so I turned to food. I gained 45 pounds during residency, and I haven't taken them off yet.

A monkey model that drives cortisol up is called the variable foraging demand model, which is the animal equivalent to "food insecurity."[11] In this model, monkeys have access to food in one of three ways: (1) ad lib, in which the food is available all the time; (2) at every meal, the animal has to work to find food that has been hidden in a maze of tubes; or (3) a random combination of the two, called variable foraging. Despite the fact that the animals in the second group have to work at finding their food, their body weights and cortisol levels are similar to those of the ad lib monkeys: they know what they have to do to attain their next meal. However, for the third group, the variable foragers, the uncertainty of the food availability drives up their cortisol levels and they become markedly obese.

Stress and cortisol also promote faster addiction to various drugs of abuse and likely food as well. Experiments in animals emphasize that stress or cortisol administration (particularly uncontrollable stress) increases the likelihood of abusing drugs such as cocaine. Another way to drive up cortisol in monkeys is by placing them in group housing, thereby exposing them to social hierarchy. Invariably, one animal will rise in the social order to become the alpha male, or the leader of the cage. This animal, akin to an all-powerful CEO, will have the lowest cortisol levels. The cortisol levels of

the subordinates will be much higher. When all the monkeys are then provided access to cocaine for self-administration, while the alpha male won't
get hooked, the subordinates become addicts. This can also happen with
food. Thus the stress and reward systems are linked, making food addiction
among those who eat to manage their stress a *faît accompli.*

Cortisol and Insulin: The One-Two Punch to Your Gut

In both rats and people, when cortisol goes up, insulin does, too. After all,
if cortisol makes you eat, your insulin levels will rise to drive the consumed
energy into fat tissue. So is cortisol the energy intake hormone and insulin
the energy storage hormone? Does cortisol have effects on obesity that are
different from those of insulin? Or are the two always yoked together? Are
their effects redundant or synergistic? These are not just academic points;
they are crucial issues in the decision tree on how to go about preventing
and treating obesity.

The only way to answer these questions is to control each hormone
separately. You can't do this in humans, but you can in rats. In a truly heroic
set of experiments, my University of California, San Francisco colleagues
James Warne and Mary Dallman answered this question beautifully.[12] In
short—insulin makes you gain weight, while cortisol tells you where to put it.
They do different things to your food intake and your fat cells (see chapter 8),
but they synergize to make metabolic syndrome worse (see chapter 9).

Cortisol and Metabolic Syndrome

There are boatloads of evidence that humans are more stressed today than
we were thirty years ago. These stresses occur at home, in the workplace,
and at school; in other words, all people all the time. Stress (e.g., job stress),
depression, and excess cortisol are all linked to metabolic syndrome. For
instance, psychosocial stresses correlate with risk of myocardial infarction
(heart attacks) in adults. One of the hallmarks of metabolic syndrome is
excessive cortisol due to adrenal gland overactivation. These examples all

suggest that cortisol is a primary player in the development of metabolic syndrome (see chapter 9).

Deconstructing Darwin

Why should cortisol lay down fat in the abdomen, where it is more likely to cause disease (see chapter 8), as opposed to your love handles? Our stressed ancestors sometimes needed lots of energy very fast, to escape the lion or to battle their neighbors. Belly fat breaks down into fatty acids faster, and has a direct line to the liver for burning. So having some extra energy that you could "mainline" right into your liver was adaptive, when the stresses were physical. Nowadays, however, stress is anything but physical, and now that abdominal fat is a liability rather than an asset.

The Limbic Triangle: Disordered Eating, Obesity, and Disease

These three brain pathways (hunger, reward, stress) drive hyperinsulinemia (excess insulin levels), resulting in obesity and metabolic syndrome (see chapter 9). We call this model the "limbic triangle"—similar to the Bermuda Triangle: once you get in, you can't get out.[13] Chronic insulin action at the VMH inhibits leptin signaling, which is interpreted as starvation. This decreases SNS activity (sloth) and increases vagal activity (hunger). In the VTA, chronic insulin deregulates hedonic reward pathways by inhibiting leptin signaling (reward). You want to eat more, especially high-fat and high-sugar treats, which results in excessive energy intake. Chronic activation of the amygdala increases levels of cortisol (stress). By itself, this promotes excess food intake and insulin resistance, ratcheting up insulin levels and accelerating weight gain.

This is what is going on in virtually every obese individual. Hunger, reward, and stress conspire to undo attempts at weight loss. The behaviors of "gluttony" and "sloth" are very real, but they are results of changes in brain biochemistry. And as you will see in part 3, these behaviors are also a result of the biochemistry of the fat cells that drive their growth.

PART III

"Chewing" the Fat

Chapter 7

The Birth, Care, and Feeding of a Fat Cell

———————●———————

Kay is a seven-year-old girl who was born at a normal weight. She first visited the clinic at age two, when she was 45 pounds (twice normal size) and her BMI was 30 (double the normal BMI for her age). Her mother and sister are both rail-thin. Lab testing showed massive insulin release, similar to that in the brain tumor children. Kay's mother kept her from all problem foods and promoted exercise as much as she could, but without effect. Over the next five years, Kay tried diet and exercise, and various weight-loss medications. Nothing seemed to slow down her weight gain. At age seven, she weighed 140 pounds, and she had a fatty liver, lipid problems, and hypertension. As a last resort, she had a lap-band procedure, to reduce her stomach's capacity. She was our youngest patient to undergo bariatric surgery at the time. Within six months post-op she had lost 30 pounds, and her face was now separate from her neck. All her labs improved. Her mother was ecstatic, in no small part because Kay could now wipe her own behind.

Your Fat, Your Fate?

In a nutshell, your body fat is your biggest long-term risk for infirmity. Nothing correlates with diabetes, heart disease, and cancer better than your fat. So is your fat your *fate*? Everyone says, "Lose the fat to extend and improve your life," but virtually no one can do it. So how do you lose the fat? Better yet, how do you prevent it from arriving in the first place, and preferably leave your muscle mass in place? In order to answer these questions a little more knowledge is required about what causes fat accumulation.

Each of us starts out as a single cell, the product of the fertilization of a sperm and an egg. As an adult, we end up having a total of between 5 and 10 trillion cells, with more than 250 cell types in our bodies. Where did the fat cells come from and why are they there in the first place? How do you make an adipocyte (fat cell)? What drives its proliferation? Can you make fewer, and would you even want to? Once a fat cell is made, how do you fill it? Finally, for all the marbles, once a fat cell is filled, how do you empty it?

These are the questions that drive scientists and the pharmaceutical industry in their quest to relegate obesity to the dustbin of medical oddities (and make a bundle in the process). The sad thing is, here we are, thirty years into the obesity pandemic, and we haven't yet harnessed the science to help us.

How Do You Make a Fat Cell?

The size of your fat tissue depot depends on two properties: fat cell number and size. In reality, the number of fat cells you have dictates your ultimate fate after they have been created. Once made, fat cells want to be filled. Think of a fat cell as a balloon. When empty, it is pretty small and many can be stored in a bag without taking up much space. The fat content is what blows the balloon up; when many are put together, they can fill an entire room. So to control obesity, you need only control your fat cell number. Alas, this is easier said than done. How and when do fat cells get born? In the early 1970s, Jules Hirsch, at Rockefeller University, demonstrated that your fat cell number is determined by age two. More recently, research has confirmed that while there is a constant low-level turnover, the majority of fat cells are formed very early in life.[1]

Why do we even need fat cells? The flippant answer is that without them, girls would look like boys. The evolutionary answer is that fat cells are repositories of energy and are necessary for survival of the species, especially in times of famine. Fat cells are protective; they provide cushioning of vital organs. In addition, specialized fat cells provide heat after you're born, to keep you from succumbing to the elements. Fat cells are not just storage devices. They are active participants in, and are necessary for, your metabolic health. As you will see in chapter 8, you need your fat cells. Fat cells are the difference between being the picture of health and suffering a miserable, lingering death.

What makes one person fatter than the next? How is it that Kay and her sister—children raised in identical environments with the same parents, values, and meals—can be so physically different from each other? Why does one child dream of nothing but soccer while the other obsesses over doughnuts? Everyone thinks they are in control, but the reality is they aren't. No one is. So please, people, give up on this idea that you are in control of your fat cells. They were laid down a long time ago. Control over your fat is an illusion promulgated by the weight-loss and fashion industry to keep you in tow, paying big bucks. Your mother was more likely in control before you were born, and she didn't even know it. (Another reason to blame Mom at the therapist's office, as if you needed one.)

Over the last twenty-five years, birth weight has increased worldwide by as much as 200 grams (half a pound), coincident with the obesity pandemic.[2] Is this conferring the risk for obesity on the newborn? It is likely that maternal weight gain is translated into fetal body fat; the more weight mothers gain during their pregnancy, the greater the birth weight of the newborn;[3] and the more fat cells early on, the greater the health risk later on.[4] Mom can bestow a blessing or a curse; what she does and eats during her pregnancy can result in an altered destiny—either way, for better or for worse.

Your fat cell number is determined before you're born and is dictated through four separate physiological pathways, none of which can you alter now.

1. *Genetics*. When we talk about genetics, we mean a change in the sequence of our DNA. Scientists routinely say that obesity is 50 percent

genetics (nature) and 50 percent environment (nurture). We do know of a few genetic mutations in the energy balance pathway that clearly predetermine your risk, which accounts for about 2 percent of morbid obesity. However, despite exhaustive searches, not that many people have genetic mutations to account for their obesity. Researchers worldwide have scanned the human genome and have identified thirty-two genes that are associated with obesity in the general population.[5] Altogether, these genes explain a total of 9 percent of obesity. And even if one person had every single bad gene variation, it would account for only about 22 pounds— hardly enough to explain our current obesity pandemic. Lastly, the genetic pool doesn't change that fast, so the gene argument can't explain the last thirty years. All these investigations show that we need to look past genetics as a cause of obesity.

2. *Epigenetics.* Epigenetics is different from genetics. It refers to changes in the areas around our genes that can cause them to be turned on or off, usually inappropriately, and that over time can result in the development of various diseases. Think of epigenetics as the On-Off switch attached to the dimmer of your living room chandelier. The gene is the light bulb; the epigene is the light switch. If the light bulb is defective or the switch is frozen in the Off position, the dimmer function is useless as it is, as it is constantly giving off low light and you are unable to read. Likewise, epigenes control the extent to which the gene turns on.

Epigenetics has become a very hot area of investigation. Here are four reasons why you should care. First, an epigenetic alteration can cause as much havoc as a genetic alteration, but the actual DNA sequence remains unchanged, so even with a full genome analysis, you can have defective epigenetics without knowing it. Second, epigenetic changes usually occur after conception but before birth. You are not just the product of your genes; you are equally the product of your epigenes. Third, changes in maternal nutrition or altered physical stress to the mother are felt by the fetus through the placenta. They can modify gene expression and function, affecting the child for the rest of his life. Fourth, and the most ominous fact of all: once your epigenetic pattern has changed, there's a better-than-even-money chance that you will transmit this same epigenetic change to your offspring, and they to theirs, *ad infinitum*. A recent study demonstrated that the epigenetic marks that babies harbor in their DNA at birth predict their degree of fat accumulation at age nine years,[6] suggesting that what the fetus experiences through the placenta has a huge impact on future risk of obesity.

3. *Developmental programming.* A relatively new field in medicine is known as developmental origins of health and disease (DOHaD), or developmental programming. We now assume that a hostile intrauterine environment (undernutrition, overnutrition, or maternal stress) transmits some signal to the fetus, which conveys information about future threat: *It's a tough world out there, kid; best be ready for it.* This drives the infant to store extra energy and increase its fat after birth when there is no need to do so, to the ultimate detriment of health later on. Such a baby's intrauterine and postnatal environment are mismatched. The child is "programmed" for survival at the expense of longevity.

David Barker first postulated that prenatal biological influences could affect postnatal outcomes for obesity. He observed that maternal nutrition affected the fetus. Small-for-gestational-age (SGA) infants (very small at birth) were at an increased risk for future obesity, diabetes, and heart disease.[7] This finding was corroborated by the Dutch Famine Study.[8] At the end of World War II, for a four-month period, the official daily rations in the Netherlands were between 400 and 800 calories per person. Those who were undernourished as fetuses developed obesity and metabolic syndrome (see chapter 9) in middle age.

Several studies of SGA newborns demonstrate that they exhibit rapid catch-up growth in the early postnatal period and develop obesity, persistent insulin resistance, and metabolic syndrome in childhood. An analysis of newborns born in Pune, India, versus those born in London demonstrated that, despite the fact that those born in India weighed 700 grams less at birth, their insulin levels were markedly elevated. After adjustment for birth weight, the India-born babies demonstrated increased adiposity, four times higher insulin, and two times higher leptin levels than their London-born counterparts.[9] Because these babies were already insulin and leptin resistant at birth, they were predestined to develop obesity and metabolic syndrome.

Worse yet, premature babies also manifest insulin resistance.[10] It's assumed that some aspect of prematurity leads to alteration in developmental programming. This is often compounded by well-meaning pediatricians, who prescribe high-calorie formula to rapidly increase the baby's weight gain. The infant is then at enormously high risk for metabolic syndrome in childhood or in adulthood.

But the converse is also true. Babies born large for gestational age (LGA) also end up with obesity and metabolic syndrome in later life.[11] They're also hyperinsulinemic and insulin resistant, but for a different reason. Most babies are LGA due to gestational diabetes mellitus (GDM), a type of diabetes that occurs in approximately 5 percent of pregnant women. The high blood glucose of the mother leads to high blood glucose of the fetus, and high insulin levels, which drive fat cells to grow. These GDM babies have three times the chance for obesity and diabetes in later life. In general, the "vertical" transmission of diabetes from mother to child has been documented in studies of the Pima, a Native American tribe in Arizona. Clearly, this is the "gift that keeps on giving."

However, GDM isn't required to produce obesity. LGA babies without GDM also have double the chance of insulin resistance and metabolic syndrome. Animal studies show that both fetal undernutrition and overnutrition can change epigenetics, making it less likely that beta-cells (cells in the pancreas that make insulin) will keep dividing. LGA children have a limited insulin reserve. As they gain weight over their lives, diabetes will be the final outcome. But this can be prevented: obese women who underwent bariatric surgery between their first and second child reduced both the chance of LGA in the second child and the second child's future risk for obesity. Fix the mother, fix the offspring.

Why does this happen? Generally, as the fetal brain develops, the hormone leptin (coming from the fetal fat cells) tells the hypothalamus to develop normally, defending against obesity. However, either lack of leptin (as in the undernourished SGA baby) or insulin antagonism of leptin action (seen in SGA, GDM, LGA, and premature babies) may prevent normal hypothalamic development and generate a baby whose brain never gets the right signal. His brain always sees starvation! The infant will eat more and exercise less right from birth, which will predispose him to obesity in later life, especially given our current overabundant food supply.[12]

4. Environmental toxins. Lastly, there is the possibility that toxins in our environment are programming increased fetal adipose tissue development. Numerous compounds in our environment, called obesogens, can act on three molecular switches to turn on fat cell differentiation. Early fetal exposure may increase the "adipocyte load," fostering future obesity, even if the exposure is short-lived (see chapter 15).

What these four lines of reasoning tell us is that the major determinant for your disease risk is the development of your fat cells before you were even born. You had no say in the matter. This can happen due to problems in the fetal liver (insulin resistance), fetal brain (leptin signaling), or the developing fat cell itself, increasing your fat cell number and storage capacity. So does this mean it's a done deal? Do all children like Kay need surgery to lose weight? Are we completely powerless to control our fate? Should you stop reading this book and live on French fries with ice cream because you are doomed anyway? Not quite.

How Do You Fill a Fat Cell?

So our number of fat cells is predetermined, but what about filling them? This is the crux of the book and the pivot on which your long-term health can turn. We could easily put our blinders on and recite the old adage that "fat cells get bigger because we eat too much and exercise too little." And, of course, we do. One recent report determined that increased caloric intake accounts for the entire U.S. obesity epidemic.[13] Alternatively, less energy expenditure, due to increased screen time and decreased physical education in schools, has been directly correlated with both obesity and the prevalence of metabolic syndrome in adolescents. Aside from the obvious changes in the caloric and exercise milieu in which we find ourselves, numerous other processes have been proffered as examples of environmental change, such as sleep debt, changes in ambient temperature, and exposure to obesity-causing viruses. Even social networks have been implicated as causes of obesity.[14]

Would that it were that simple. All these are examples of correlation, not causation. The journey through obesity and chronic metabolic disease begins and ends with the hormone insulin, the energy-storage hormone (see chapter 4). There is no fat accumulation without insulin. Insulin shunts sugar to fat. It makes your fat cells grow. The more insulin, the more fat, period. While there are many causes of obesity, excess insulin (known as hyperinsulinemia) in some form is the "final common pathway" for the overwhelming majority of them. Block it, and the fat cells remain empty.

And we're all making more insulin than we used to. Today's adolescents have double the level of insulin secretion of their predecessors in 1975.[15] High insulin is responsible for perhaps 75–80 percent of all obesity.

There are three different ways to increase your insulin:

1. If, in response to a meal, particularly one high in refined carbohydrates (see chapter 10), your pancreas makes extra insulin (called insulin hypersecretion), it will drive your fat cells to store energy.[16] This happens when your brain sends a signal to the pancreas through the vagus, or "energy storage," nerve.

2. If, because of the specific foods you eat (see chapters 9 and 11) you build up fat in your liver, this fat will make the liver sick (called insulin resistance). The pancreas has no choice but to make more insulin in order to force the liver to do its job. This raises insulin levels throughout the body, driving energy into fat cells everywhere, and making other organs sick as well.

3. If your stress hormone cortisol (which comes from your adrenal gland) increases, two things will happen. It will work on the liver and muscle to make them insulin resistant, raising your insulin and driving energy deposition into fat. It may also work on the brain to make you eat more (see chapter 6).

Of course, these three insulin problems are not mutually exclusive. One person could have more than one problem going on at a time, which makes it even harder to diagnose and treat.

There's yet another way that our current society increases insulin and weight gain. Three classes of medicines (steroids to control inflammation, antipsychotics to stabilize mood, and oral hypoglycemic agents to treat diabetes) are notorious for driving insulin up and causing excessive weight gain. Bottom line, once a glucose molecule is in the bloodstream it has one of three fates: it can be burned (by exercise), it can be stored in fat (by insulin), or it can be excreted in the urine (which eventually kills your kidneys). It's way better not to need these drugs in the first place—but usually they are the lesser of two evils.

Can You Get Your Fat Cells to Slim Down?

As you can imagine, these biochemical pathways are pretty darn powerful. Fat cells want to be downsized about as much as General Motors or AIG. And it doesn't matter if you're young or old—your fat is here to stay. Once the balloon is filled, it doesn't want to be deflated. It's because of insulin that weight loss is so difficult. Virtually every aspect of our modern society drives our insulin levels higher and higher. From an evolutionary perspective, our ancestors had to work hard in the face of famine to accumulate their fat. Their children needed to be prepared for this fate *in utero* to have a chance at survival. Once the fat is stored we don't want to give it up, at least not without a fight. Because when fat cells get smaller, they stop making leptin. And when there's no leptin, there's no puberty, no pregnancy, no human race. To add insult to injury, our current drug armamentarium is only minimally effective in promoting fat loss (see chapter 19).

So, how do we slim down a fat cell? What options are left? One promising research tool is to deprive fat cells of their blood supply. Investigators are actively pursuing the possibility of using chemicals called angiogenesis inhibitors, which would cut off the blood supply to fat tissue. Animal experiments using these compounds demonstrate melting away of the fat tissue. But it will be years before we are ready for trials in humans. Other compounds are in development, but likewise it will be a long time before they're ready to use. In fact, many drug companies have left the obesity research business, despite the promise of the pot of gold at the end of the rainbow (see chapter 19).

So, at least today, there's only one hope: Reverse the biochemistry. Stop the energy storage. Fix the leptin resistance. Lowering the insulin works on both counts. But there are two problems with this strategy:

First, not everyone has the same insulin problem. So giving general guidelines is not going to work for everybody. We need some version of "personalized obesity medicine." Second, changes in the environment are what drive the biochemistry. If you want to fix the biochemistry, you have to fix the environment. And that's not easily done. Parts 5 and 6 will provide some guidance.

Chapter 8

The Difference Between "Fat" and "Sick"

———————•———————

July 21, 2009, abcnews.com
"Critics Slam Overweight Surgeon General Pick,
Regina Benjamin" —By Susan Donaldson James

"Dr. Regina M. Benjamin, Obama's pick for the next surgeon general, was hailed as a MacArthur Grant genius who had championed the poor at a medical clinic she set up in Katrina-ravaged Alabama. But the full-figured African-American nominee is also under fire for being overweight in a nation where 34 percent of all Americans aged 20 and over are obese.

Even some of the most reputable names in medicine chimed in. 'I think it is an issue . . .' said Dr. Marcia Angell, former editor of the *New England Journal of Medicine* . . . 'It tends to undermine her credibility . . . at a time when a lot of public health concern is about the national epidemic of obesity, having a surgeon general who is noticeably overweight raises questions in people's minds.'"

Even Dr. Angell, an intelligent woman by any definition, doesn't get it. Do you think Dr. Benjamin chose to be obese? Do you think she's a glutton and a sloth given her talents, character, and track record? Is she overweight? Sure. Is she sick? Don't bet on it.

Most people in the modern world do not want to be thought of as obese. Here's a politically incorrect disclosure: my pediatric colleagues and I see Latino mothers who come to clinic with infants whose weights top the charts and tip the scales. And these women are worried, but in the opposite direction. "*No come*" (Spanish for "He doesn't eat"), they moan. There is a racial/ethnic overlay to obesity. This is in part due to societal norms and what's expected for your culture. For instance, some extremely poor countries have developed a set of cultural norms that equate obesity with affluence and desirability. Fatty foods, such as meat and dairy, were scarce in their native countries, and pitifully available only to the wealthy. Upon moving to America, immigrants from developing countries are suddenly immersed in a glut of rich energy-dense foods, and they overindulge as their insulin increases. Sometimes these cultural views persist throughout generations. The immigrants view their obese children as the epitome of health and an affirmation of their ability to provide for them. In their countries of origin, thin children were sickly and at risk of premature death. Unfortunately, they aren't yet familiar with the fact that the opposite is true in America.

More political incorrectness: some teenage African American girls tip the scales at 300 pounds, but when you ask them if they think they're obese, many will say, no, that they're "thick" (which describes a girl who isn't fat or skinny, but is well proportioned, and has meat on her bones and in all the right places). Many DJs still play Sir Mix A Lot's song, "Baby Got Back," "I like big butts and I cannot lie. . . ." (Those of you with young children and not hip with modern tuneage may instead recognize this song as sung by the character Donkey in *Shrek*.) Then again, it's long been known that, when polled, women consistently underestimate their weight. (Don't worry ladies, you're not alone in the exaggeration department; men consistently overestimate their height and other lengths as well.) Clearly obesity, like beauty, is in the eye of the beholder.

There seems to be a genetic component to this as well. Several studies have looked at how much fat must be present before signs of illness develop. And the results are striking, if not surprising. Caucasians start showing metabolic wear and tear at a BMI of around 30, which is why epidemiologists chose 30 as the obesity breakpoint. However, African Americans don't show metabolic decompensation until a BMI of about 35, while Asians start to manifest disease at a BMI of around 25.[1] On average, an African American woman can carry an extra 27 pounds over an Asian female (half of which is fat, half muscle), before she can expect some kind of negative impact from that extra weight.

Many of my patients will say to me, "As long as I feel all right, my weight's not a problem." They may very well be right. But for how long? Which brings us to an important precept about body weight. Whenever we step on the scale, we are measuring the sum of four different body compartments, only one of which is bad for us.

1. *Bone.* The more bone, the longer you live. When little old ladies fracture their hips, that's their swan song. African Americans, to their benefit, have a greater bone density than do other races.

2. *Muscle.* More muscle is better for your health. Muscle takes up glucose. More exercise means more muscle, and more muscle means better insulin sensitivity. Arnold Schwarzenegger in his weightlifting days (anabolic steroids or not) had a BMI of 32, not because he was obese but because he was all muscle and had very little fat. When you're building bone and muscle, you are providing a method for burning energy rather than storing it, which leads to improving your health regardless of your weight.

3. *Subcutaneous (or "big butt") fat.* This makes up about 80 percent of our total body fat and is what gave Marilyn Monroe her hourglass figure. Believe it or not, more subcutaneous fat is better for your health. Several studies show that the size of the subcutaneous fat depot correlates with longevity. Little old ladies who don't have much subcutaneous fat get sicker and die sooner, and not just from their hip fractures.

4. *Visceral fat.* The only compartment that is consistently bad for us is our visceral (aka abdominal, ectopic, or "big belly") fat. This consists of fat in areas where it doesn't belong, including fat inside your abdomen and inside your organs (e.g., liver and muscle). It makes up about 20 percent of our total body fat, or about 4–6 percent of our total body weight. Visceral fat is the fulcrum on which your health teeters.

The Scale Lies Even More Than You Do

Not all pounds are created equal. The scale lies—you were right all along!—at least in terms of your health and your lifespan. In fact, the majority of Americans now have a BMI of over 25, which puts them in the overweight category. Studies show that, on average, people with a BMI of 25–30 have the longest lifespan.[2] So being overweight is good? Yes, all you Kate Moss wannabees—provided the weight is in the right place.

Do you ever wish that all the fat on your body would somehow miraculously disappear? That some talented plastic surgeon could painlessly remove every cubic centimeter of unwanted adipose? For free and with no lasting scars or cellulite? Come on, admit it. It's a recurrent dream of virtually everyone on the planet. Even men.

Think again. What would life be like without any fat? Pretty damn miserable, and short to boot. Indeed, some unfortunate souls get to experience this firsthand. It's called lipodystrophy and it's one of the worst diseases known to humankind.[3] It can be genetic or acquired as a complication of AIDS therapy. With it, you look weird, gaunt, and as if you're circling the grave, which you are. When your body wants to store energy, there's no place for it to go. So it goes to the only places it can—your liver, muscles, and blood vessels. The organs of people with lipodystrophy get filled with fat and they develop diabetes, hypertension (high blood pressure), and heart disease.

Bottom line, you need your fat. At least you need your subcutaneous or "big butt" fat, which provides a bucket for extra energy to keep you alive and healthy. With rare exceptions, your subcutaneous fat contributes very little to the development of chronic disease. Twenty percent of morbidly obese adults have completely normal metabolic status, no evidence of disease, and normal longevity. In fact, the smaller your subcutaneous fat compartment, the faster you die.

When it comes right down to it, it's all about your middle. This whole obesity/health/longevity question centers on your abdominal, visceral, or "big belly" fat—at least statistically. All this hoopla about one body compartment, which constitutes only 4–6 percent of your total weight. But it translates into the difference of about fifteen years of life.[4] Here, size really does matter; it means dying in your fifties of a heart attack or cancer versus living into your eighties or longer. Visceral fat depots are more metabolically active than subcutaneous fat depots, and they drive inflammation. Visceral fat causes insulin resistance, which in turn promotes diabetes, cancer, cardiovascular disease, dementia, and aging. While the populace is more worried about subcutaneous fat (because it's unsightly), this fat is much less prone to being lost; in fact, it is rarely shed unless you go on a caloric restriction or starvation diet, which is rarely sustainable.

It's the visceral fat that doctors care about, because it's the visceral fat that kills you. When you lose weight on any diet, it's the visceral fat that is lost first. It's there for easy access for energy (see chapter 6), so it's the first to go. And that's good. But your body defends its subcutaneous fat, because that's the fat that makes leptin, and your body (your brain) knows it's good for you. And it's even more specific than that. Your visceral fat is really just a proxy for your "ectopic," or intra-organ, fat—the fat in your liver and muscles. This is the real killer. But it is too hard to measure without very specialized imaging techniques such as MRI or liver ultrasound. Chronic metabolic disease starts when fat deposits itself in organs such as muscles and especially the liver.

This fact is borne out in a recent study comparing BMI to percentage body fat by X-ray methods. It appears that many as 50 percent of women and 20 percent of men who are categorized as normal on the basis of their BMI are actually obese based on their carriage of visceral (bad) fat.[5] The study's author, Dr. Eric Braverman, called BMI the "Baloney-Mass Index," because it gives a false sense of security to those who follow it. Indeed, Dr. Jimmy Bell of London, using MRI scans of the abdomen, realized that body size is irrelevant; it's visceral fat that drives disease. He coined the expression "thin on the outside, fat on the inside," or TOFI.[6] Bottom line, it's your visceral fat, in particular your liver fat, that counts.

How Do You Measure Visceral Fat?

Standing on a scale is great for determining your wrestling weight class, but it is woefully inadequate for just about any other purpose. It is particularly useless for discerning how healthy you are or whether you are at risk for metabolic disease and/or death. BMI is problematic because, as a measurement, it can't distinguish between the four body compartments of bone, muscle, subcutaneous fat, and visceral fat. Doctors use BMI anyway because it works at a population level, but not necessarily for their individual patients. The reason is that, excluding African Americans (like Dr. Benjamin), who get five extra BMI points for free, and the 20 percent of obese subjects who are metabolically normal, if your BMI is over 30 you likely have a significant visceral fat component and some level of metabolic dysfunction.

Still, we need a better measure than BMI of where your body fat is located, how much, and what it means. The simplest and cheapest surrogate for determining your health status is your waist circumference, which correlates with morbidity and risk for death better than any other health parameter.[7] This is arguably the most important piece of information in your entire health profile because it tells you about your visceral fat. A high waist circumference translates into the "apple" shape that tips physicians off to risk for diabetes, heart disease, stroke, and cancer. But physicians are loath to measure this in the office because you need a metal tape measure, the measurement is subject to error, different people do it differently (the two sanctioned methods use completely different body landmarks), it takes time and effort, and it means getting "up close and personal" with the patient. Furthermore, the doctor often doesn't know what to do with the results except say, "You should really eat less and exercise more."

A reasonable proxy is belt size. Greater than 40 inches for males and 35 inches for females is a likely indicator of visceral fat, which is correlated with insulin resistance and risk for metabolic disease in adults[8] and in children.[9] But you can imagine that people who wear their pants way below their beer belly might get the measurement wrong. As long as you have someone to help you, you might also try to measure your hip circumference. A waist-to-hip ratio of greater than 0.85 (in women) or 1.0 (in men) is another warning sign of insulin resistance, versus a waist-to-hip ratio of 0.8 or less, which suggests metabolic normalcy. Waist circumference is more complicated to measure and determine in children because it is dependent on sex, age, and race. While standards have been published, none of the childhood obesity guidelines from any of the medical societies currently advocate using waist circumference as a screen for metabolic disease.

Another simple method for determining your metabolic status is to look at the back of your neck, armpits, and knuckles. What you're looking for is acanthosis nigricans, or a darkening, thickening, and ridging of the skin. Many people think this is dirt or, in the case of the neck, "ring around the collar," but it's actually excess insulin working on the skin (the epidermal growth factor receptor, to be exact). You might also see skin tags in these areas. Both of these are visible signs of insulin resistance and predict future risk for chronic metabolic disease. Every other method to find out your metabolic risk is expensive and requires blood drawing, specialized equipment, and professional data analysis.

Weight Loss Is the Wrong Approach and the Wrong Outcome

Any doctor will tell you that losing weight will improve your health, including me. And it's a fact—except for two small problems: First, weight loss is next to impossible. Witness all the money wasted on weight-loss aids. And second, it's only half-true. (See, even I lie!) When you go on a diet to lose weight, what are you losing? You lose some fat, but you're actually losing more muscle, unless you exercise while you're dieting in order to prevent the muscle loss. Remember, muscle is good for you. Even if you lost subcutaneous fat easily, it wouldn't help your health. A group of obese women were studied before and after liposuction, which vacuums out subcutaneous fat only. Their metabolic status didn't improve despite an average 20-pound weight loss.[10] So aside from not being easy, losing weight is a bit of a crapshoot in terms of effectiveness.

And here's the catch-22 of weight loss: thanks to the DEXA scan (an X-ray method of determining body composition), we know that when you lose subcutaneous fat (the fat underneath the skin) by dieting, you also lose an equal amount of muscle. Your percentage of fat stays the same. A decidedly good-news, bad-news deal.

So what should your doctor be telling you? No question, if you're obese and you want to improve your health, you want to lose some fat. But the fat you want to lose is the visceral, or the ectopic (intra-organ, as in liver) fat. If you lose subcutaneous fat, too, that's a bonus. Your doctor will tell you that losing even 5 percent of your body weight will be beneficial, which is true. Because that 5 percent is likely going to come from your vis-

ceral/ectopic/metabolically active fat. If you are obese, the National Institutes of Health recommends losing 7–10 percent of your body weight to
reduce your risk of life-threatening illness.[11] I agree; just make it your visceral fat—that's the key to improving your individual health outcomes.
Watch your waist circumference. If your pants fit better, then you are
healthier. But if you think you're going to be able to lose that big butt with
any rational diet, think again. You might be able to do so—for a short time.
But as you lose subcutaneous fat, and your leptin levels fall, your brain will
sense starvation, and reduce the activity of your sympathetic nervous system (see chapter 4), reduce your energy expenditure, make you feel lousy,
and activate your vagus nerve. Viva Las Vagus! That darn vagus will drive
up your appetite, your insulin, and energy storage to replace what you lost.
And you're going to regain the visceral fat first. Screwed yet again.

So how can anyone do it? What's rational? What's effective? What
strategy will improve your health? If I didn't think this could be accomplished, I wouldn't have bothered writing this book. The short answer is
that it depends on how you got there in the first place. Because obesity isn't
one disease; it's many. This isn't a one-size-fits-all deal. Like anything in
medicine, different problems require different approaches. As you saw in
chapters 4–6, there are three reasons to eat—two insulin problems and one
cortisol problem—and they all have different solutions. These solutions will
be discussed in detail in chapters 17–19. The short answer is that to get
your visceral fat down, you don't necessarily need to lose weight. But you
will have to do something different.

Chapter 9

Metabolic Syndrome: The New Scourge

———————●———————

Diana is an eight-year-old Latino girl who weighs 200 pounds. Despite not yet starting puberty, she has already been diagnosed with type 2 diabetes. For the past two years, she and her mother have lived in a homeless shelter. The child constantly cries for food despite being given ample portions. To feel that she can provide for her daughter, her mother also gives Diana her own portion of every meal served by the shelter. Worse yet, Diana gets a third breakfast at the school as part of the USDA School Nutrition Program. While Diana's mother does what she feels is in the best interest of her daughter, she is inadvertently making her sicker and likely contributing to an early death.

The numbers don't lie: the fatter you are, the quicker you die. At least at a population level. An actuarial analysis in 2003 demonstrated that those with a BMI of 45 lost a total of twenty years of life.[1] As a rule, the fat die young. Ford now makes cars specifically suited for the obese in America, and we've even super-sized our caskets. But we're talking statistics for large populations of people here. At an individual level, all bets are off. Twenty percent of the obese population have a normal metabolic profile, whereas up to 40 percent of normal-weight people have an abnormal metabolic profile. Knowing where you stand is crucial to taking steps to prolong your life.

Metabolic Syndrome

You don't die of obesity; you die of the diseases that "travel" with it. It's these metabolic decompensations that make obesity the scourge that it is. Diabetes, hypertension, heart disease, cancer, and dementia—the things that kill you are collectively packaged under the concept of "metabolic syndrome."

Metabolic syndrome is classically defined by the National Cholesterol Education Program's Adult Treatment Panel (NCEP-ATP) as a cluster of five chronic conditions (obesity, diabetes, lipid problems such as high triglyceride and low HDL, hypertension, cardiovascular disease), any or all of which increase your chance of early death. The NCEP states that if you've got three of the five, you've got metabolic syndrome. However, the syndrome is not nearly so easy to define. Other professional organizations have chosen to define it using slightly different criteria.[2] The reason for these alternate diagnostic benchmarks is that we really don't know the true cause. All the benchmarks try to establish cutoffs, which are fraught with error. Establishing criteria for metabolic syndrome in children is even more difficult.[3] But it's crucial, because the problem is increasing at alarming rates and translates into fifteen to twenty years of life lost. Metabolic syndrome may soon overtake smoking as the leading cause of heart disease worldwide.

The concept that cardiometabolic risk factors "cluster" in certain individuals has been known for several decades. However, it was not until the early 1980s that the relationship between obesity, dyslipidemia (an abnormal amount of cholesterol and/or fat in the blood), and hypertension was recognized. Only then did the roles of insulin resistance and abdominal obesity become apparent. But metabolic syndrome should be considered a spectrum of diseases. And not all the diseases hit each person; it tends to be "mix and match."

Racial/Ethnic/Sex Differences in Metabolic Syndrome

Males with metabolic syndrome are seven times more likely than females with metabolic syndrome to have nonalcoholic fatty liver disease (NAFLD). Race is one of the biggest determinants of what diseases you are susceptible to. For example, blacks do not get the hypertriglyceridemia (high levels of triglycerides in the blood; see chapter 10) that Caucasians do, but they tend to have higher blood pressure levels independent of body weight. Hence, despite having higher rates of diabetes and cardiovascular disease, blacks are diagnosed with metabolic syndrome less frequently. Conversely, Latinos have an increased prevalence of hypertriglyceridemia, but they have less hypertension. Hispanic males are approximately seven times more likely to have the diagnosis than non-Hispanic males. Blacks and Latinos also appear to be more insulin resistant than Caucasians. All these data reinforce the fact that racial/ethnic/sex differences in metabolic syndrome and its components make it very hard to use hard-and-fast cutoffs for its diagnosis.

How Insulin Resistance Becomes Metabolic Syndrome

You don't have to be obese to have metabolic syndrome. After all, up to 40 percent of normal-weight adults have it! Obesity is a "marker" for metabolic syndrome, but not the only marker; it is not the cause. Whether it resides in fat people or not, the one thing everyone seems to agree on is that insulin resistance is the hallmark of metabolic syndrome. And thin people can be insulin resistant, too. But how? And where? And why does the body become insulin resistant? Here is one postulated scheme by which metabolic syndrome occurs[4]:

1. Metabolic syndrome starts as your body accumulates energy, storing it in the liver and in visceral fat tissue. This makes the liver insulin resistant, which starts metabolic dysfunction—a detrimental cascade of effects that damages every organ in the body.
2. Liver insulin resistance causes the liver to transport energy improperly. The pancreas responds by increasing insulin release to make the liver do its job. This drives insulin levels even higher (hyperinsulinemia), which causes further energy deposition into subcutaneous fat tissue and causes the persistent weight gain that drives obesity.

3. The liver tries to export the excess fat as triglycerides, to be stored in the subcutaneous fat tissue. The blood lipids rise to drive dyslipidemia (see chapter 10), one of the risk factors for heart disease.
4. The high insulin acts on blood vessels, causing the smooth muscle cells that surround each blood vessel to grow more rapidly than normal. This process tightens the artery walls and promotes high blood pressure.
5. The combination of insulin resistance, lipid problems, and high blood pressure wreaks havoc throughout the body. This promotes cardiovascular disease, which can result in heart attack or stroke.
6. The fat in the liver causes inflammation, which drives further insulin resistance. Eventually the liver can scar, which results in nonalcoholic fatty liver disease (see chapters 11 and 14). This can later progress to cirrhosis.
7. Insulin resistance and hyperinsulinemia in women can drive the ovary to make extra testosterone and reduce estrogen, resulting in polycystic ovarian syndrome, hirsutism (excess body hair), and infertility.
8. As the liver insulin resistance gets worse and the body fat grows, the pancreas has to make more insulin. Eventually the pancreatic beta-cells can't keep up with the body's requirements, which leads to a relative insulin deficiency. Eventually the beta-cells fail, precipitating type 2 diabetes.
9. Insulin is one of the hormones that cause cells to divide. Hyperinsulinemia is associated with the development and growth of various forms of cancer.
10. There is early evidence, although by no means proven, that insulin resistance in the brain leads to dementia.

Basically, the various diseases of metabolic syndrome are where virtually all our health care dollars are going. So understanding these disease processes is essential for making any headway in our current health care debacle.

The First Hit: The Liver Dilemma

Under normal circumstances, approximately 20 percent of your caloric intake goes to the liver. The liver uses that energy for three tasks. First, it burns some of it for its own metabolism and livelihood. Second, when the energy source is glucose (the major energy source of all living things, and the building block of complex carbohydrates), the liver turns the excess glucose into glycogen (liver starch), stimulated by the hormone insulin. Glycogen is the storage form of glucose in the liver. Glycogen isn't dangerous; it provides us with a ready supply of glucose should we need it. Third, the liver has to deal with excess energy, which may arrive in several forms: as fatty acids from digestion of dietary fat or as amino acids from the digestion of protein, the consumption of alcohol, or from the molecule fructose (which is half sucrose, or table sugar, and roughly half high-fructose corn syrup). This extra energy is processed by the liver into fat. The liver needs to transport this fat out, or it will muck up the works. If it can't, the liver can get very sick, very fast. Bottom line: in the liver, glycogen is good, fat is bad. And anything that drives liver fat accumulation, even in children such as Diana, is a potential driver of metabolic disease (see chapters 10 and 11).

The Second Hit: Reactive Oxygen Species (ROS) and Disease

Okay, that's one problem. What else drives metabolic dysfunction? And in so many tissues? Glucose is the preferred energy source of all organisms on the planet. If you don't consume glucose, your liver will make it out of what's available. Glucose metabolism occurs through two distinct pathways. The first is called glycolysis, which converts glucose into the energy intermediate pyruvate, liberating a small amount of energy. The second step is called the Krebs cycle. It occurs within the mitochondria (the cell's equivalent of a coal furnace), and burns the pyruvate down to carbon dioxide and water, liberating a lot of energy in the process. About 80 percent of energy intake will be metabolized in this way. When your body burns energy, some toxic metabolites (breakdown products of a reaction) get manufactured within the mitochondria; these are called reactive oxygen species (ROS). They are the body's equivalent of hydrogen peroxide. In some parts of the body, ROS are put to good use. For instance, when found within your white blood cells, ROS are part of your body's immune defense system to kill foreign invaders so you don't get infected.

But ROS are also by-products of normal energy metabolism. When they are made in other types of cells, such as those of the liver or pancreas, they can do damage to the cells' DNA, proteins, or membranes. ROS require the help of antioxidants to quench them before they have a chance to do damage. That is the function of another part of the cell, called the peroxisome, which is full of antioxidants. Most of these come from the foods you eat in the form of micronutrients (see chapter 14). Peroxisomes live right next to mitochondria, and act as the "mop-up crew" for excess ROS. When the peroxisomes can keep up with the ROS generated inside the cell, you and your cells stay healthy. When they can't, the cell either is damaged or dies. These two hits together cause the cell to crap out, and when enough cells give up, you've got the basis for metabolic syndrome.[5]

The Four Foodstuffs of the Apocalypse

Many investigators have spent considerable resources searching for the gene or genes that cause metabolic syndrome. As with obesity, the genetic analyses have thus far been unrevealing. In fact, it has been suggested that only about 10 percent of metabolic syndrome can be explained by genetics.[6] This leaves approximately 90 percent to changes in the environment, specifically the quality and quantity of our food intake, and how these promote liver insulin resistance.[7]

When the energy bolus comes as glucose (starch), the liver has several safety mechanisms, including letting the other organs deal with it (spread the pain), and conversion to glycogen, keeping the liver safe. But when the liver has to deal with foodstuffs that can't be metabolized by other organs, the result is the excess production of ROS and liver fat, which gets transported out as triglycerides (blood fats) (see chapter 11). When energy supplies overwhelm the mitochondria's ability to handle them, the result is a buildup of ROS and fat deposition in the liver ("mitochondrial constipation," if you will), leading to chronic metabolic disease. These foodstuffs tend to affect different age groups based on their frequency in the American diet. What foodstuffs have this unique signature to cause this metabolic disturbance? There are four, by my count.

1. *Trans fats.* These can't be broken down by the mitochondria because of their synthetic nature.[8] Trans fats have long been assumed to contribute to chronic metabolic disease, especially atherosclerosis (hardening of the arteries). Trans fats used to be in every processed food, although slowly they are leaving our diet. But they are still in baked goods and candy bars. In fact, any food in a wrapper at room temperature that's meant to sit on a store shelf is suspect. The FDA and the food industry have since recognized the problem that trans fats pose, and while there is no nationwide ban on them, there is currently a concerted effort to remove them from our diet. For instance, Mayor Michael Bloomberg has banned the use of trans fats within restaurants in New York City. Yet, despite the cutback on trans fats, the rates of obesity and diabetes continue to rise.

2. *Branched-chain amino acids.* These are essential amino acids, meaning our bodies cannot make them so they must be eaten in our diet. Blood levels of branched-chain amino acids are directly related to consumption. These amino acids are in high concentration in corn, so every animal fed on corn (e.g., U.S. beef and pork) is a potential contributor to your total body load. While these amino acids are necessary for building proteins all around the body, any in excess are burned for energy in the liver. Body builders consume these with abandon in their protein powders, and as long as these people are building their bodies, no problem. For everyone else, however, big problem. When branched-chain amino acids are metabolized for energy, they bypass glycogen in the liver and go straight to the mitochondria for burning, or to be turned into fat (see chapter 10). Christopher Newgard at Duke University has demonstrated that patients with metabolic syndrome exhibit higher levels of these amino acids in the bloodstream.[9] But at this point, we only have correlation, not causation.

3. *Alcohol.* Alcohol is interesting because a small daily ration, especially when consumed as wine, has been shown to *prevent* metabolic syndrome. (If you have high cholesterol, your doctor may recommend a glass

or two of red wine with dinner.)[10] But increased consumption of booze clearly contributes to metabolic syndrome's development. Furthermore, alcoholic beverages that also contain glucose, such as beer and shochu (a Japanese fermented drink) have been clearly implicated in the promotion of metabolic syndrome in America and Japan, respectively.[11] Alcohol also goes to the mitochondria without stopping at glycogen. However, alcohol certainly does not explain how children get metabolic syndrome or why metabolic syndrome is rampant in alcohol-abstaining Muslim countries such as Saudi Arabia and Malaysia.

4. *Fructose.* Finally, we come to the Voldemort of the dietary hit list: the sweet molecule in sugar. If it's sweet, and it's caloric, it's fructose. Period. This is the one foodstuff whose consumption has increased worldwide, and with reckless abandon. And it is the one that children eat with no holds barred. We have animal and human data. We also have the golden ticket: correlation *and* causation. Every age group, including infants, has increased its consumption of fructose in the last thirty years. As far as I am concerned, this is where the action is, and will be fully elaborated in chapter 11.

Can't We Just Pop a Pill?

In a word, no. There's no drug target to stop this process, because ROS formation is a fact of life. We've got medicines that can treat the various downstream outcomes. We have statins and fibrates for lipid problems; antihypertensives to reduce blood pressure; insulin and other hypoglycemic agents to treat diabetes; loads of drugs to make the heart beat better and stronger; vitamin E and metformin for fatty liver; dialysis and transplantation for chronic kidney disease; various chemotherapies once you get cancer; and even new Alzheimer's drugs. But your mitochondria are still screwed. And the lipogenesis and ROS damage will continue unabated. Your cells will die, and so will you. But you and Diana aren't doomed. You can slow the process down considerably.

The easiest and most rational approaches to reducing ROS formation and toxicity are preventive. You can: limit specific substrate availability (modify your diet; see chapters 11, 17, 18); reduce the rate at which the liver metabolizes energy (eat more fiber; see chapter 12); increase your antioxidant capacity (consume micronutrients; see chapter 14); and/or increase mitochondrial formation and number to improve mitochondrial capacity and efficiency (exercise; see chapter 13). We're talking altered intake and expenditure. If you've overindulged your entire life, and you want to get on the bandwagon now, all is not lost. Studies of patients with diabetes who improve their lifestyle (e.g., eat properly and exercise) demonstrate reduction in total body burden of ROS, improved health, and increased longevity.[12]

Oh no! Diet and exercise again! Is this whole book just a crock? Why did I spend good money for the same message? Didn't I already know this? No, because it's not just "eat less, exercise more." We're talking about something specific. Because *a calorie is not a calorie.*

PART IV

The "Real" Toxic Environment

Chapter 10

The Omnivore's Curse: Low Fat versus Low Carb

———————•———————

Sally is a beautiful thirteen-year-old girl, but since the age of eleven she had been gaining 20 pounds per year. She has the lead in her middle school musical and is mortified because she can't fit into her costume. She comes to my clinic after her family's attempts at lifestyle intervention are ineffective. An oral glucose tolerance test shows that her pancreas releases too much insulin (see chapter 19), yet she is also insulin resistant and glucose intolerant. We place her on a low-carb diet and prescribe metformin (see chapter 19) to lower her insulin. She loses 20 pounds in the first three months, another 10 pounds after that, and holds steady thereafter. She isn't abnormally hungry anymore, and her insulin levels have returned to normal. She is a very happy camper.

The "Hunters"

In the beginning there were the hunters. Most hunters killed their food, while some fished. They ate fat and protein, went long stretches between kills, and had to live off their fat stores. Their livers processed dietary fat in one of two ways based on the hunters' body weight and their current energy supply. If energy was in short supply, the liver would chop up the fatty acids (long carbon chains) systematically into 2-carbon fragments called acetyl-CoA, or ketones. These fragments could then be burned for energy either by the mitochondria (the portion of the cell where energy generation occurs), in the liver, or in other organs. If the energy supply was in excess, the liver would package the fat into particles known as low-density lipoproteins (LDL). These LDL particles would circulate in the bloodstream and eventually take up residence in fat cells to be stored as triglyceride (blobs of fat) for another day, when energy might be needed when food was scarce. In the absence of insulin (as would occur in starvation), this stored triglyceride would break down into free fatty acids. The cycle would then repeat itself—the stored triglyceride would be released into the bloodstream, re-enter the liver, and be chopped up into 2-carbon fragments to make acetyl-CoA, or ketones, again. These hunters didn't know what a carbohydrate was and they didn't need to, as animal (and human) carcasses were devoid of carbohydrates. Our bodies were, and are, perfectly adapted to burning fat as an energy source.

This is the nature of what has become known as the low-carb diet. Natural examples of this can still be found in cultures around the world, such as the Maasai and Samburu tribes of north-central Kenya (who eat meat, milk, and animal blood) and the Inuit of the Arctic (who eat fish, meat, and whale fat). In the early 1900s, the Arctic explorer Vilhjalmur Stefansson (1879–1962) lived among the Inuit for several years, subsisted primarily on whale blubber, and never felt healthier. He was the first to note that the Inuit, who ate nary a carbohydrate, had an extraordinarily low incidence of cancer, heart disease, diabetes, and other chronic diseases. (This has unfortunately changed in recent years with the introduction of processed foods into their diet.) When he returned to the United States in the late 1920s, Stefansson undertook an experiment. Under medical supervision, he ate only meat for one year and was documented to have no negative health effects from his diet. Stefansson wrote the 1960 book *Cancer: Disease of Civilization?* about his experiences and observations.

The low-carb diet has achieved mythic status. In the 1970s, Dr. Robert Atkins transformed it into high art—cheeseburgers without the bun, bacon and eggs, and broccoli with cheese sauce. No toast or potatoes, and woe to the beer drinkers. It continues to recruit record numbers of followers, who swear by it for treatment of obesity and promotion of health. The low-carb movement hit its peak in 2002, with the publication of two *New England Journal of Medicine* articles demonstrating its utility.[1] Die-hards still swear by it, mainstream obesity experts have gotten on the bandwagon, and the number of positive testimonials can be documented with one click of your mouse. But in the recent past, the low-carb diet has come under fire, as it is very difficult to stay on it in America. It has also been criticized for having potential negative health impacts.[2]

The "Gatherers"

Alongside the hunters, there were the gatherers. The gatherers found their food in what came out of the ground. They ate carbohydrates and proteins in the form of fruits and vegetables. If energy was in short supply, the glucose would be completely taken up by the liver. If the gatherers' energy status was instead replete, the liver would not capture some of the glucose and a rise in the blood glucose and subsequent insulin release would occur. If energy was in great surplus, then the blood glucose would rise even higher and insulin would keep pace, driving energy into fat for storage for a rainy day (e.g., famine).

This is the basis for today's vegan diet. It is practiced in multiple cultures around the globe, because if you grow your own food, that's what's available. Many people in the United States eat this way as a matter of choice and sometimes to an extreme. (For example, fruitarians eat only fruits, nuts, and seeds, and some fruitarians eat only that which has naturally fallen from the tree, to avoid hurting the plant.) This diet can also be perfectly healthy and, when practiced properly, lifesaving.[3]

The Omnivore's Curse

The conflict between these two dietary philosophies is touched on in Michael Pollan's 2006 book *The Omnivore's Dilemma*. Evolutionarily, the metabolism of fat and carbohydrates developed separately. The net energy recoupment of each of these processes is minimal. But both metabolic products of these two completely different pathways (fat being broken down serially versus carbohydrates undergoing glycolosis) meet at the mitochondria in the form of the compound acetyl-CoA. As we learned in chapter 9, how much acetyl-CoA the mitochondria have to process has *everything* to do with how healthy the cell is. It also determines whether the cell will collapse under the weight of processing all that energy.

The hunters ate fat; the liver would beta-oxidize (the process by which fatty acids are broken down by the mitochondria, two carbons at a time) what it needed for its use and would then export any excess LDL to be taken up in adipose tissue. The gatherers ate carbohydrates (glucose); after absorption, the liver would extract what it needed and the insulin would clear the rest out into the bloodstream for muscle and adipose tissue. In the liver, any excess glucose would be converted to glycogen for storage. Our ancestors were rarely exclusively hunters *or* gatherers, but they likely favored one food type (fat or carbohydrate) over the other depending on where they lived and the time of year. The liver thus developed two separate pop-off valves to protect it from excess energy, one for carbohydrate and one for fat. In both cases, the mitochondria's exposure to acetyl-CoA was exquisitely regulated so as not to overwhelm their capacity. The mitochondria never had to bite off more than they could chew.

But then, as humans learned to irrigate and farm, we became omnivores. Sally, and with few exceptions, our entire society, eat fat and carbohydrates at the same meal (e.g., steak and potatoes). As food became more plentiful, we began to overload both sides of our metabolic pathways: the 2-carbon breakdown of fat *and* the glycolysis of carbohydrates. Now the mitochondria are catching hell; they have to deal with an onslaught of acetyl-CoA coming from both directions. One high-fat, high-carbohydrate meal is no big deal. But keep this up for ten thousand meals in a row (about ten years; just in time for your teenage years) and we're talking about some real damage: an increase in chronic metabolic disease or metabolic syndrome.

Fat *or* Carbohydrate? Or Fat *and* Carbohydrate?

Here's some food for thought. With very few exceptions, every naturally occurring foodstuff contains either fat *or* carbohydrates, but usually not both. Meat, fish, and poultry have no carbohydrates. Grains, roots, and tubers (e.g., potatoes and yams) have no fat. Those fruits that have fat, such as avocados, olives, and coconut, have minimal carbohydrates. Nuts are an exception, but they are still pretty low in carbohydrates and very high in fiber. (That's why they're brown; see chapter 12.) Milk is another exception to the rule, but other than that which came from their mothers, humans were not exposed to other mammals' milk until the beginnings of agriculture, in the Neolithic period. They didn't have a USDA Food Pyramid to follow.

It wasn't until we became *gourmets*, eating fat and carbohydrates in the same meal, that our cells first felt the wrath of mitochondrial wear and tear. This accounts for the appearance of metabolic disease with the advent of trade in the early seventeenth century; before that, food was still a function of what you killed or you grew yourself. Eventually, we became *gourmands*, eating fat and carbohydrate in the same food. This is the essence—the blessing and the curse—of processed food. Except for one big item, which has both fat and carbohydrates at the same time. (I'll give you a hint: it's really sweet.)

The Battle Royale

The prevalence of heart disease had begun to rise slowly over the early twentieth century when Paul Dudley White wrote his classic treatise *Heart Disease* in 1931. White was Eisenhower's cardiologist in 1955 after the president's heart attack. The move to reduce heart disease through dietary intervention was in full swing by the 1960s, with the U.S. government wanting to take a proactive role. This set the stage for a nutritional "holy war," played out in kitchens and restaurants across America. The goal was to alter our diet for the better. Instead, we've laid waste to every nutritional hypothesis, lost the public's trust, and killed countless millions in the process. We will be suffering the aftermath of this Battle Royale for generations to come.

The first salvo in the battle emanated from the dental community. Prior to 1960, the known problems associated with sugar were restricted to the development of cavities.[4] With the advent of water fluoridation in 1945, cavities were no longer a public health issue. Sugar dropped from the radar.

Enter John Yudkin and Ancel Keys. Yudkin, a British physiologist and nutritionist, researched the nature of chronic disease. In 1957 he postulated that dietary composition was the cornerstone of coronary thrombosis (heart attacks). By 1964 he had determined through natural observation that the consumption of sucrose was most closely associated with heart disease. He was the first to show that sugar uniquely raised serum (blood) triglycerides and insulin levels. In 1972 he published his seminal work on the subject, *Pure, White, and Deadly,* in the United Kingdom. Yudkin published countless papers on the biochemistry of sucrose, specifically the molecule called fructose, which gives sugar its sweetness. He was the first to warn that excessive consumption could lead to coronary heart disease, diabetes, GI disease, eye disease, and other inflammatory diseases.

Ancel Keys, a Minnesota epidemiologist, was already in the public eye as the inventor of the K-ration during World War II. In 1952 he took a sabbatical in England, where he saw enormous increases in heart disease in the face of the English diet, which consisted of incredibly high fat and high cholesterol items. (Think bangers and mash, fish and chips.) He noted that those who were the best fed in both the United States and the United Kingdom, those able to afford meat, were the ones who suffered most often from heart problems. He returned to the United States on a mission to prove that cholesterol and dietary fat were the direct sources of heart disease.

Keys published many studies in the 1960s and '70s that demonstrated higher cholesterol levels in patients with heart disease; he also showed that increased consumption of dietary fat led to higher cholesterol. Keys' seminal "Seven Countries" study (1980) was a 500-page volume dedicated to the concept that, through its cholesterol content, dietary fat was the single cause of heart disease. Unfortunately, based on his own work, there are four problems with his thesis.

1. The Seven Countries study started out as the Twenty-two Countries study. Keys' seven countries were Japan, Italy, England, Wales (included as a separate country by Keys), Australia, Canada, and the United States. For these seven, the relationship between dietary fat and heart disease looked pretty convincing. But when all twenty-two countries were plotted (add Austria, Ceylon, Chile, Denmark, Finland, France, Germany, Ireland, Israel, Mexico, Netherlands, New Zealand, Norway, Portugal, Sweden, and Switzerland), the correlation became a lot less convincing. He also chose to leave out "indigenous tribes," such as the Inuit (North America), Tokelau (Oceania), and Maasai and Rendille (both Africa), who ate only animal fat and have among the lowest prevalence of heart disease on the planet.

2. The role of dietary fat in heart disease is complicated by the consumption of trans fats (e.g., margarine), which are a significant factor in the etiology of metabolic syndrome. Trans-fat use peaked in the 1960s with the advent and popularization of margarine—remember Imperial Margarine, "fit for a king"?—just as Keys was starting his epidemiologic research. Could he have been studying an effect of trans fat instead of saturated fat in the developed countries? Since he did not separate the two in his work, we don't know.

3. The correlation itself is a problem. At one end of the graph are Japan and Italy, as they eat the least amount of saturated fat. But they also eat the least amount of dietary sugar of all the countries included. How can you determine whether it is the fat or the sugar that is driving this relationship when both go together?

4. On page 262 of his mega-opus, Keys wrote, "The fact that the incidence rate of coronary heart disease was significantly correlated with the average percentage of calories from *sucrose* in the diets is explained by the intercorrelation of sucrose with saturated fat." In other words, sucrose also correlated with heart disease, but Keys did not think this was an issue. When one does a multivariate correlation analysis (determining whether A causes B regardless of the impact of C, D, and E) one has to do it *both ways*; in this case, one would need to hold sucrose constant and show that dietary fat still correlates with heart disease. Keys didn't perform this kind of analysis. We don't know why. So which was it—the fat or the sugar?

Kick It up a Notch, and BAM . . .

In the midst of the Yudkin-Keys battle came the lipid hypothesis of heart disease. In the 1970s, the Nobel Prize–winning team of Michael Brown and Joseph Goldstein in Dallas discovered how the liver recycled fatty acids.[5] From this discovery we learned four important precepts. First, we identified LDL, or low-density lipoproteins (the main export particle of dietary fat), and the liver LDL receptor (which gobbles them up to recycle them). Second, we learned that dietary fat increased blood LDL levels. Third, one rare genetic disease generates massively high LDL levels, and these patients die of heart attacks very early in life. Fourth, in large populations of adults, blood LDL levels correlate with risk for coronary heart disease.

The implications of this work seem quite logical on the surface. Let's call dietary fat A, LDL B, and cardiovascular disease C. The implication was that "If A leads to B, and B correlates with C, then A must lead to C; therefore, no A, no C."

This was the debate of the late 1970s, specifically taken up by Senator George McGovern's bipartisan, nonlegislative Select Committee on Nutrition and Human Needs in 1977, and chronicled by Gary Taubes.[6] McGovern appointed a labor reporter named Nick Mottern, who had no scientific background, to research and write the first dietary goals for the United States. Rather than doing extensive research on the subject, Mottern relied almost exclusively on the work of Mark Hegsted, a nutritionist at the Harvard School for Public Health. Hegsted was of the opinion that dietary fat was the ultimate cause of dietary woes in the United States, and that the solution was to limit its intake. Thus, Mottern's report recommended that the American populace limit its fat intake to 30 percent of their diet and saturated fat to 10 percent. Mottern admitted that not all scientists agreed with his suggestions, but he stated that Americans could only improve their health by following his advice. What did they have to lose?

Although it took seven years and several twists and turns, the USDA, the AHA, and the American Society of Clinical Nutrition all endorsed the document. Mottern's brainchild, *Dietary Goals for the United States*, was implemented, and our dietary practices began to change as the food industry retooled itself to deliver low-fat products rushed to meet the new directives.

What Went Wrong?

Seems logical—A to B to C; so no A, no C—i.e., no dietary fat, therefore no LDL, and no heart disease. Not so fast. A can lead to B, but it can also lead to D, E, F, and G, and never make it back to C. And the contrapositive of the statement is, "No C, no A." This is flawed logic, to be sure.

The implicit assumption was that all LDL was bad. As it turns out, there are *two* types of LDLs: one is called large buoyant LDL, or type A LDL, and the other is called small dense LDL, or type B LDL. Large buoyant LDL floats in the bloodstream. It's too big to get underneath the cells lining your blood vessels to start the atherosclerotic (artery wall thickening) process. Eighty percent of blood LDL is large buoyant and is thought to be neutral from a cardiovascular standpoint. However, small dense LDL doesn't float; it sinks. It's small enough to get underneath the blood vessel cells and has been specifically implicated in the start of atherosclerotic plaques. True, dietary fat raises LDL, but it's the large buoyant kind. The small dense variation is raised by carbohydrates.[7]

Here's one more fly in the ointment. Dietary fat isn't one entity. It's at least seven, listed in table 10.1. Some of these, such as omega-3 fatty acids, are good for you and protective against heart disease. Trans fats are disasters because our mitochondria can't break them down completely for energy. Because *a calorie is not a calorie*. The fat remnants precipitate in arterial walls—a great way to get a heart attack. Omega-6 fats are pro-inflammatory and associated with heart disease. Keys' personal demon was saturated fat, which is in the middle of this spectrum and does neither harm nor good. Indeed, recent studies have exonerated saturated fat from a primary role in the atherogenic process.[8]

Table 10.1. Dietary Fats and Their Value,
in Descending Order, to Human Health

Dietary Fat	Dietary Source	Medicinal Value or Danger
Omega-3 fatty acids	Wild fish, flaxseed oil	Anti-inflammatory, lowers serum triglycerides, repairs membranes
Monounsaturates	Olive and canola oil	Stimulates liver metabolism, reduces atherogenesis
Polyunsaturates	Vegetable oils	Anti-inflammatory, but in excess amounts can cause immune dysfunction
Saturated fatty acids	Grass-fed animal meats, milk and dairy products	Atherogenic in a specific genetic background (familial hypercholesterolemia, or FH); raises levels of type A LDL very high
Medium-chain triglycerides	Palm oil, coconut oil, palm kernel oil	Energy source, some suggestion of stimulation of atherosclerosis
Omega-6 fatty acids	Farm-raised animals and fish (fed on corn and soy)	Atherosclerosis, insulin resistance, immune dysfunction, pro-inflammatory
Trans fats (partially hydrogenated oils)	Synthetic, found in processed foods only	Atherosclerosis, nonalcoholic fatty liver disease

But the proof's in the low-fat pudding, right? Does a low-fat diet prevent heart disease or not? This was put to the test in the Women's Health Initiative, started in 1993. The study followed nearly fifty thousand postmenopausal women over eight years. Fat (saturated, monounsaturated, and polyunsaturated) was decreased in their diets to 30 percent of their total calories—but there was no change in the incidence of heart attack or stroke. A long-term, prospective, randomized controlled study on a lot of people, and it was a bust.[9]

The Devolution of Our Diet

Nevertheless, in the early 1980s, none of these concerns about sugar, carbohydrates, and types of fats was known. With the endorsement of the *Dietary Guidelines*, Keys delivered the knockout punch and won the food fight, while Yudkin was thrown under the bus. We were beseeched to reduce our consumption of dietary fat from 40 to 30 percent. The food industry had to retool its products to meet the demand for low-fat fare. This meant altering its recipes. But when you take the fat out, the food tastes like cardboard. And palatability equals sales. The food industry had to find ways to make this low-fat fare palatable. They therefore upped the carbohydrate content, specifically the sugar. An example is Nabisco SnackWells, which are still stocked on the shelves. For each serving, 2 grams of fat were removed and 13 grams of carbohydrates, 4 of which were sugar, were added.

In the 1990s there was a major shift in the availability of specific foodstuffs. The foods containing fat, such as milk, saw a drop or a stabilization in consumption. Conversely, levels of refined carbohydrates, devoid of their inherent fiber, went through the roof. Remember, refined carbohydrates means lots of insulin, which means more energy storage in fat tissue. And thus the obesity epidemic was born in the aftermath of this seemingly logical and well-meaning, yet tragically flawed, understanding of our biochemistry.

The gradual understanding that dietary fat isn't always the demon that it was portrayed to be in the *Dietary Guidelines*, and the work of Dr. Robert Atkins and other pioneers, led to the introduction of the "low-carb diet" into the American lexicon. Restaurants started serving cheeseburgers wrapped in a lettuce leaf instead of a bun (hold the fries). By the early 2000s, the carbohydrate-restricted diet was put to the test; it went head to head against the low-fat diet for the treatment of obesity and type 2 diabetes. From controlled studies, we learned the following five lessons[10]: First, carbohydrate restriction improves glucose control, the primary target of diabetes therapy. Second, carbohydrate-restricted diets are at least as effective for weight loss as low-fat diets. Third, substitution of fat for carbohydrates is generally beneficial for markers of and incidence of heart disease. Four, carbohydrate restriction improves features of metabolic syndrome. Five, the beneficial effects of carbohydrate restriction are independent of weight loss. (Look at Sally.) Carbohydrate restriction lives on in many guises throughout the food world. Yet so do the vegan, traditional Japanese, and other low-fat, high-carbohydrate diets.

Because the two overlap.

There is one specific foodstuff that is both fat *and* carbohydrate at the same time. It's the one item that's excluded from every successful diet in the world. It the *real* omnivore's curse. And it's the real culprit of the global obesity and metabolic syndrome pandemic.

Chapter 11

Fructose—The "Toxin"

———————●———————

Gabriel is a 100-pound eight-year-old boy who has mildly elevated blood pressure. His father is a type 2 diabetic and has already had a gastric bypass. A dietary analysis of the family's eating habits exhibits no abnormalities, *except* that the father is a truck driver for the Odwalla juice company and is allowed to bring home as much product as he wants. Gabriel's mother limits her son to one glass of juice per day, but he admits to drinking three glasses per day. We counsel the parents to remove juice from the house. Within one year, the father loses 20 pounds and his diabetes improves, while Gabriel has not gained any weight and his blood pressure has returned to normal.

The Fructose Epidemic

Can low-fat and low-carb diets *both* be right? Or *both* wrong? What do the Atkins diet (protein and fat), the Ornish diet (vegetables and whole grains), and the traditional Japanese diet (carbohydrate and protein) have in common? On the surface they seem to be diametrically opposite. But they all have one thing in common: they restrict sugar. Every successful diet in history restricts sugar. Sugar is, bar none, the most successful food additive known to man. When the food industry adds it for "palatability," we buy more. And because it's cheap, some version of sugar appears in virtually every processed foodstuff now manufactured in the world. Sugar, and specifically fructose, is the Lex Luthor of this story.

Nutritionists routinely categorize sugar as "empty calories," interchangeable with calories from starch. But sugar has a special payload. Sugar (sucrose) is made up of half glucose and half fructose. It's the fructose that makes it sweet, and that, ultimately, is the molecule we seek. It's the fructose that causes chronic metabolic disease. So sugar, despite ostensibly being a carbohydrate, is *really* both a fat (because that's how fructose is metabolized in the liver) and a carbohydrate (because that's how glucose is metabolized) all rolled into one. Both pathways have to work overtime, which is why sugar is the real omnivore's dilemma. Now, if you're starving and energy-depleted, consuming sugar can replete your liver's glycogen stores more rapidly, which can be beneficial. So offensive linemen after three hours on the gridiron can consume all the Gatorade they want. But the overwhelming majority of people are neither starving nor energy-depleted (there are now 30 percent more obese individuals than undernourished ones on the planet). Our bodies have not adapted to our current environmental sugar glut, and it is killing us . . . slowly.

Fructose has increased both as a percentage of our caloric intake and our total consumption. When you add it up, Americans currently consume sugar at a rate of 6.5 ounces a day, or 130 pounds a year. Our current fructose consumption has increased fivefold compared to a hundred years ago, and has more than doubled in the last thirty years.[1] A recent survey by the CDC estimates that 50 percent of Americans have one can of sugared soda per day, and 5 percent of Americans have four or more.[2] In other words, we're not just eating more—we're increasing both the amount of sugar we eat, and sugar as a percentage of our daily caloric allotment. The inescapable reality is that 20–25 percent of all the calories we consume, a total of twenty-two teaspoons per day, comes from some variation of sugar.[3] And some adolescents are consuming 40 percent of their calories as sugar. This can't be good for you.

Okay, America is sugar-dipped and candy-coated. But that's not true elsewhere—or is it? World sugar consumption has tripled in the last fifty years, while the population has only doubled. That means our global per capita intake of sugar has increased by 50 percent, commensurate with this pandemic. The upper threshold of 200 calories per day of sugar, advocated by the American Heart Association in its scientific statement for optimal cardiovascular health,[4] has been exceeded in virtually every country on the planet.[5] This is a massive increase from just thirty years ago, when most countries were bereft of sugar.

When reading the title of this chapter, your first reaction may be "Aha! I knew it! High-fructose corn syrup is evil." You're half right. Media attention and consumer activist groups have started to vilify HFCS due to its synthetic nature and assumed effect on the obesity epidemic. As a result, its consumption has been declining since 2007. But our rates of obesity remain unchanged. HFCS is ubiquitous in the United States and Canada, but it is used more sparingly in the European Union and Japan. The rest of the world uses sucrose. Australia and the entire Pacific Rim, for example, have only sucrose, but they are right behind us in terms of obesity and metabolic syndrome. Scientific studies of acute satiety versus energy intake and of metabolic alterations support the notion that HFCS is technically no different from sucrose, although HFCS does generate a higher blood fructose level, which could have negative metabolic consequences.[6] This has led to a vociferous campaign by the Corn Refiners Association, and its public commercials, arguing that HFCS is a natural, out-of-the ground, and benign sweetener. HFCS is biochemically similar to "natural" sucrose (made of glucose and fructose), taking "corn syrup" (glucose) through an enzymatic process so that approximately half the glucose becomes fructose, in order to make it sweeter. The question is not whether HFCS is worse or better than sugar; the question is whether sugar (in any of its forms) is *toxic*?

The health-conscious among you may opt for juice over soda. For those of you who can afford it, you skip the Sunny Delite in favor of "natural 100 percent fruit juices" made by Odwalla or other organic companies. They tout multiple health benefits and claim that, because they are devoid of added sweeteners, they are in fact good for you. Wrong. The fruit is good for you, because it also contains fiber (see chapter 12). In fact, calorie for calorie, 100 percent orange juice is worse for you than soda, because the orange juice contains 1.8 grams of fructose per ounce, while the soda contains 1.7 grams of fructose per ounce.

All caloric sweeteners contain fructose: white sugar, cane sugar, beet sugar, fruit sugar, table sugar, brown sugar, and its cheaper cousin HFCS. Add to this maple syrup, honey, and agave nectar. It's all the same. The vehicle is irrelevant; it's the payload that matters. Bottom line, sugar consumption is a problem, 33 percent of sugar consumption comes from beverages, and the biggest abusers are the poor and underserved.

A Carbohydrate Is a Carbohydrate—or Is It?

All carbohydrates are not created equal. Just as there are different grada-tions of fats (see chapter 10), there are different gradations of carbohydrates based on their metabolism.[7] To illustrate how this works, consider the fol-lowing exercise involving the metabolism of three different carbohydrates of equal caloric value (120 calories): glucose, ethanol (grain alcohol), and fructose.

Glucose

Despite its absolute necessity for life (see chapter 10), dietary glucose isn't perfect. When it exists in nature without fructose, it's called "starch," and it truly does supply "empty calories," energy for either storage or burning. But the Atkins, Paleo, and caloric-restriction adherents will all tell you that the glucose molecule has three metabolic downsides, all of which do damage over time and necessitate the limitation of its consumption. To demonstrate this, let's consume 120 calories of glucose (e.g., one-half cup cooked white rice). Twenty percent, or 24 calories, will enter the liver, whereas the rest will be metabolized by other organs in the body. Here's what happens:

1. Glucose metabolism is insulin-dependent. Consuming glucose raises the glucose level in the bloodstream, stimulating insulin release, which promotes energy storage into fat cells and causes weight gain.
2. The overwhelming majority of glucose in the liver will be directed toward forming glycogen, or liver starch, which is not harmful to

the liver cell. This also will keep the liver from releasing glucose into the blood, preventing diabetes.

3. A small amount of glucose will be metabolized by the liver mitochondria for energy.

4. Any excess glucose in the liver that is not shunted to glycogen and not metabolized by the mitochondria for energy will instead be converted to triglycerides. High triglyceride levels in the blood can promote development of cardiovascular disease.

5. Glucose can bind to proteins in the cell, which causes two problems:

   • When glucose binds to proteins throughout the body, the proteins become less flexible, contributing to the aging process and causing organ dysfunction.

   • Every time a glucose molecule binds to a protein, it releases a reactive oxygen species (ROS; see chapter 9), which can cause tissue damage if not immediately mopped up by an antioxidant in the peroxisome (see chapter 14).

Like all things, glucose in excess can be bad for you—especially when it lacks fiber, which limits the insulin response (see chapter 12). However, you would have to consume a lot of it and over a long period of time for glucose to have these detrimental effects. In general, large amounts of glucose (starches such as pasta, white bread, rice, etc.) will cause you to gain pounds but it won't make you sick. Rather, if over time you gain too much weight from glucose, the visceral fat that is formed will eventually take its toll on your health (see chapter 8). But when you consume the same number of calories as either ethanol or fructose, you get much more of a bang to your liver (more like a hand grenade), and it takes its toll that much faster.

Ethanol (Grain Alcohol)

Ethanol is a naturally occurring by-product of carbohydrate metabolism, called fermentation. Upon ingestion of 120 calories of ethanol (e.g., a 1.5-ounce shot of 80-proof hard spirits), 10 percent (12 calories) is metabolized within the stomach and intestine (called the first-pass effect) and 10 percent is metabolized by the brain and other organs. The metabolism in the brain is what leads to the alcohol's intoxicating effects. Approximately 96 calories reach the liver—four times more than with glucose. And that's important, as the detrimental effects are dose-dependent.

1. After ethanol enters the liver in high dosages, it can promote ROS formation and cell damage.
2. In contrast to glucose, which went to glycogen, the ethanol goes straight to the mitochondria.
3. Any excess gets turned into fat by a process called *de novo* (new) lipogenesis (fat-making). The lipid buildup can lead to liver insulin resistance and inflammation.
4. If this process continues, it can eventually cause alcoholic liver disease. This is a surefire prescription for slow death or, at best, a liver transplant.
5. Alternatively, the lipid can exit the liver and take up residence in skeletal muscle, where it also induces insulin resistance and can cause heart disease.
6. Lastly, ethanol enhances its own consumption, by acting on the brain's reward pathway. When this goes out of control (chapter 5), addiction sets in.

Thus, for the same number of calories, ethanol is more likely than glucose to cause chronic disease.

Fructose

Fructose is never found alone in nature. Rather, it is always partnered with its more benign sister molecule, glucose. They both have the same chemical composition ($C_6H_{12}O_6$), but they are hardly the same. Fructose is much worse. Let's start with the Maillard, or "browning," reaction. This is the same reaction that turns hemoglobin in your red blood cells into hemoglobin A1c (HbA_{1c}), the lab test that doctors follow to determine how high a diabetic patient's blood sugar has risen over time. The reaction product is brown; this is the reason bananas turn brown with time and also why barbecue sauce caramelizes the meat underneath when exposed to heat. So, you can brown your meat at 375 degrees for one hour, or you can brown your meat at 98.6 degrees for seventy-five years. The result is the same. And fructose drives the Maillard reaction seven times faster than glucose.[8] This seemingly subtle difference can cause every cell in the body to age more rapidly, driving various degenerative processes such as aging, cancer, and cognitive decline.

There are dozens of studies that now implicate fructose as a major player in causing metabolic syndrome. In fact, it's metabolized a lot like ethanol. Let's now consume 120 calories of sucrose (60 of glucose, 60 of fructose)—for example, an 8-ounce glass of orange juice. (As I mentioned before, juice is just as bad as soda, if not worse.) The 60 calories of glucose do the same 20-80 split, so 12 calories of glucose will enter the liver. But, unlike with glucose, which can be metabolized by all organs, the liver is the primary site of fructose metabolism (although the kidney has the capacity to metabolize a few calories in rare cases). Give or take, the whole 60 calories of fructose end up in the liver. So, the liver gets a 72-calorie dose, triple the amount as with glucose alone.

The unique metabolism of fructose can induce each of the phenomena associated with metabolic syndrome:

1. Triple the dose means the liver needs triple the energy to metabolize this combo versus glucose alone, depleting the liver cell of adenosine triphosphate (or ATP, the vital chemical that conveys energy within cells). ATP depletion leads to the generation of the waste product uric acid. Uric acid causes gout and increases blood pressure.
2. The fructose does not go to glycogen. It goes straight to the mitochondria. Excess acetyl-CoA is formed, exceeding the mitochondria's ability to metabolize it.
3. The excess acetyl-CoA leaves the mitochondria and gets metabolized into fat,[9] which can promote heart disease (see chapter 9).
4. Fructose activates a liver enzyme, which is the bridge between liver metabolism and inflammation. This inactivates a key messenger of insulin action, leading to liver insulin resistance.

5. The lack of insulin effect in the liver means that there is no method to keep the glucose down, so the blood glucose rises, which can eventually lead to diabetes.

6. The liver insulin resistance means the pancreas has to release extra insulin, which can force extra energy into fat cells, leading to obesity (see chapter 4). And the fat cells that fill up most are in the visceral fat, the bad kind associated with metabolic disease.

7. The high insulin can also drive the growth of many cancers.[10]

8. The high insulin blocks leptin signaling (see chapters 4 and 5), giving the hypothalamus the false sense of "starvation," and causing you to eat more.

9. Fructose may also contribute to breakdown of the intestinal barrier. Normally the intestine prevents bacteria from entering the bloodstream. This intestinal breakdown may lead to a breach in the walls of the intestine. The result is a "leaky gut,"[11] which could increase the body's exposure to inflammation and more ROS. This worsens insulin resistance and drives the insulin levels even higher.[12]

10. Fructose undergoes the Maillard (browning) reaction 7 times faster than glucose, which can damage cells directly. Although the experiments are in their infancy, preliminary results suggest that in a susceptible environment, fructose can accelerate aging and the development of cancer.

11. The data on fructose and dementia in humans are currently correlative and indirect. However, the data on insulin resistance and dementia show clear causation. African Americans and Latinos are the biggest fructose consumers and those with the highest waist circumference (a marker for insulin resistance). Coincidentally, they also have the highest risk for dementia.

Fructose versus Ethanol: Pick Your Poison

Studies of alcohol use show that a little bit is good for you. Alcohol raises HDL (good cholesterol), and red wine has the compound resveratrol, which is thought to improve insulin sensitivity and longevity (see chapter 14). As with alcohol, a small dose of fructose has been shown in some studies to have a beneficial effect on insulin secretion. The toxic effects of fructose, just like those of alcohol, are dose-dependent. For alcohol, we have empiric evidence that in most people, a maximum dose of 50 grams per day (about three glasses of wine) is the threshold for toxicity.[13] This is likely the threshold for fructose as well (slightly less than a quart of orange juice). The problem is that the current *average* adult fructose consumption is 51 grams per day. That means that more than half the population is over the threshold.

When you look at chronic alcoholics versus those consuming massive amounts of sugar, they often appear very different, at least on the outside. Many alcoholics are thin, if puffy, compared to those consuming massive amounts of sugar. But remember, we're not concerned with subcutaneous fat. It's the visceral fat—the fat that surrounds your organs and often remains invisible to the naked eye—that's going to kill you. Both alcohol and sugar significantly increase your visceral fat and your likelihood of developing associated diseases. The difference between alcoholic fatty liver disease and nonalcoholic fatty liver disease lies only in the terminology—the effect on the body is the same.

Of course, the major difference between alcohol and sugar is alcohol's intoxicating effects; the brain does not metabolize fructose. People don't get arrested for driving under the influence of sugar. But the liver's metabolism of fructose is remarkably similar to that of ethanol. Fructose isn't the only cause of obesity, but it is the primary cause of *chronic* metabolic disease, which kills . . . slowly. Fructose can fry your liver and cause all the same diseases as does alcohol. We know we must limit our ethanol consumption or face the consequences. But sugar flies under the radar. No wonder Saudi Arabia and Malaysia have the highest rates of type 2 diabetes on the planet. No alcohol, but they're drinking soft drinks like they're going out of style.

Sugar and the Global Diabetes Pandemic

According to the International Diabetes Federation (IDF), the global diabetes pandemic currently claims 366 million people. That's a prevalence
rate of 5.5 percent of the world's population. And they're breaking the bank
on health care worldwide (see chapter 1). While it would be easy to lay the
blame on the fast food industry, whose outlets continue to propagate worldwide, lots of countries whose populations do not overindulge in McDonald's are also experiencing increases in obesity and diabetes. What's changed
in the food globally?

My colleague Sanjay Basu and I are attempting to answer that
question by looking at food supply data worldwide. The Food and
Agriculture Organization (FAO) monitors the world's food supply. FAO
keeps close tabs on food supply data, broken up by type of foodstuff. We
linked the FAO food supply database with the IDF prevalence database
and with the World Bank Gross National Income database (to control for
poverty). We are currently performing an epidemiological analysis for
154 countries around the world, known as an "ecological" analysis,
between the years 2000 and 2010. We asked two questions: Does the
increase in caloric intake per capita correlate with increase in diabetes
prevalence? And if so, is there any aspect of the diet that explains this
relationship?

In the time period we studied, diabetes prevalence worldwide rose
from 5.5 percent to 7.0 percent. Surprisingly, total calories did not correlate
with diabetes prevalence worldwide. Instead, the correlation with the percentage of calories coming from sugar and sugarcrops was enormous. For
every 100 calories supplied as sugar, the prevalence of diabetes rose by 0.9
percent, even after controlling for obesity in each country. The amount of
sugar availability explains more than one fourth of the increase in diabetes
prevalence rates worldwide during the last decade, even after controlling
for aging and obesity in the population. And those few countries whose
consumption went down experienced a reduction in diabetes prevalence of
0.18 percent. This is not *correlation*, but rather *causation*.

If you had any residual doubt about "*a calorie is not a calorie,*" this
analysis should remove it. Every additional 150 total calories per person

per day barely raised diabetes prevalence. But if those 150 calories were instead from a can of soda, increase in diabetes prevalence rose sevenfold. Sugar is more dangerous than its calories. **Sugar is a toxin**. Plain and simple.

There are clear limitations to doing this kind of analysis. First, food supply does not automatically mean consumption. However, in most parts of the world, the two are closely aligned. Only in the United States do we throw away significant amounts of food (up to 30 percent of what we produce). Second, populations are diverse, in socioeconomic status, vulnerability, and food preference. So, what you learn from a population may not be immediately ascribable to one individual. Third, estimating diabetes prevalence is always difficult. Different countries use different criteria for diagnosis, many people go undiagnosed, and the IDF pools people with type 1 and type 2 diabetes. Nonetheless, the robustness of the effect is undeniable. The global industrial diet that revels in sugar consumption clearly negatively affects the metabolic health of entire countries, unrelated to obesity.

The Sweetest Taboo: Fructose, Reward, and Addiction

Now you're thinking: diabetes, liver dysfunction, cancer, dementia, and aging—it couldn't get any worse, could it? Oh, but it can. Not only does fructose turn your liver to fat and your proteins brown, but it tells your brain that you need more of it . . . and more. Remember the starvation pathway (see chapter 4), and the reward pathway (see chapter 5)? Similar to the effects of alcoholism, fructose stimulates excessive and continued consumption by tricking your brain into wanting more. For Gabriel, one glass of juice just wasn't enough.

Fructose Drives Reward and Food Intake

Recall the lessons of leptin. Anything that blocks leptin signaling will be read as starvation at the hypothalamus (chapter 4) and as lack of reward by the nucleus accumbens (chapter 5); both of which drive long-term food intake. And anything that alters the meal-to-meal hunger and satiety signals will drive short-term food intake. When you don't feel full, you consume more. Fructose does them all.

1. Consumption of fructose does not stimulate an insulin response, so leptin doesn't rise and the animal keeps eating (or drinking soda, as the case may be).

2. Long-term fructose consumption generates liver insulin resistance and causes chronic hyperinsulinemia (excessively high blood insulin), which interferes with leptin signaling and promotes further food intake by preventing dopamine clearance from the NA (see chapter 5).

3. Ghrelin, a peptide produced by cells in the stomach, is the "hunger" signal. In humans, ghrelin levels rise with increasing subjective hunger, peak at the time of voluntary food consumption (which is why your stomach grumbles at noon), and decrease after a meal. However, fructose intake does not decrease ghrelin; therefore, caloric intake is not suppressed. Indeed, fructose consumption in the form of a Big Gulp does not reduce the volume of solid food needed to feel satiated, multiplying the total calories consumed during the meal.

Deconstructing Darwin

So why do we have this fascination with sugar in the first place? Why does sugar make us want more? What's the selective advantage? In chapter 4 we saw that insulin blocks leptin signaling to promote leptin resistance, in order to allow the weight gain associated with puberty and pregnancy to occur. In chapter 5 we saw that sugar stimulates brain dopamine and opiates to let us know what foods are safe. But why should sugar cause insulin resistance and hyperinsulinemia? Naturally occurring sugar in fruit is what makes fruit palatable. But for our ancestors, fruit was readily available for one month per year, called "harvest time." Then came four months of winter, and no food at all. We needed to stock up—to increase our adiposity in preparation for four months of famine. In other words, in the doses that were available to our forebears, sugar was evolutionarily adaptive. Indeed, fruit binges among orangutans in Indonesia are responsible for their altered energy intake and changes in weight. For their normal diet, they consume 21 percent of their calories as fruit—as opposed to when fruit is plentiful during a binge, at which point that figure rises to 100 percent. This results in high insulin, driving energy storage and cyclic adiposity.[14] But with our current global sugar glut, devoid of fiber and in high doses 24/7/365, our weight gain is not cyclic anymore, and this process has become maladaptive.

Face it, we've been "frucked."

Still, while sugar is the biggest perpetrator of our current health crisis, it is by no means the only bad guy. There are "antidotes" to the fructose effect, but they have been removed from our environment as well. The rest of part 4 will lay bare the rest of our "toxic environment."

Chapter 12

Fiber—Half the "Antidote"

———————•———————

Sujatha is a thirteen-year-old Indian girl who has just been diagnosed with type 2 diabetes. At a height of 5 foot 4 inches, she weighs 170 pounds. According to her BMI, she is technically obese, but she doesn't look it. Her mother is a nurse in a local hospital and also a type 2 diabetic. She told me, "I don't understand how this can happen. We are Indian, we are vegans at home." However, the family consumes large volumes of "white foods" such as naan, rice, potatoes, and processed starches. Almost completely lacking from their diet are "brown foods" such as lentils, garbanzo beans, and whole grain products. Like many teenagers, Sujatha refuses to eat her vegetables. Beverages consist of soda and juice, and virtually no water. The fiber content of their diet is close to zero.

The Stealth Nutrient

Fiber, also known as roughage or bulk, is the most misunderstood weapon in our nutritional arsenal. The common belief, promulgated by countless TV commercials playing to the over-seventy crowd, is that fiber is important for our bowels and little else. Fiber makes you "regular" (as if constipation makes you "erratic"?). These commercials suggest that you should start eating fiber to make those golden years a little smoother. Meanwhile, gastroenterologists have impressed upon us the value of fiber to prevent both colon cancer and diverticulitis. All that's true—but fiber is oh so much more. As you will see, fiber is half of the "antidote" to the obesity pandemic. But how can something that we don't even absorb be so darn valuable?

Unlike the other foodstuffs previously discussed—fats, proteins, and carbohydrates—fiber isn't digested or absorbed by your body. It travels through and out of your stomach, small intestine, and colon with minimal alteration. The USDA does not classify fiber as an essential nutrient; indeed, most people consider fiber a waste product of food and a waste of time. Despite this, the Dietary Reference Intake for fiber suggests a total of 14 grams per 1,000 calories, or essentially 25 grams of fiber per day.[1] Paleobiologists have performed DNA footprint analyses of three- to ten-thousand-year-old stool samples from caves in Texas, allowing them to determine what our ancestors ate based on the bacterial makeup of their intestines. They estimate that these cave dwellers consumed about 100 grams of fiber per day,[2] yet our median consumption of fiber is currently 12 grams. Does this matter? Why should we care about fiber? Why does processing a food remove its fiber? Aside from our current "irregularity," what might our lack of fiber be doing to us? After all, it's just to make us poop "regular," right?

Definitions

Dietary fiber—found in fruits, vegetables, whole grains, and legumes—is the part of the plant that the human gut is unable to digest. So, you can't use it for energy. Therefore it has one destination: the toilet. There are two types of fiber: soluble, which dissolves in water, and insoluble, which does not (see table 12.1). This difference determines each type of fiber's impact on your body, health, and stool. Soluble fiber slows digestion and absorption, and is fermented by the bacteria of your colon into gases (read: socially unacceptable emissions except for teen boys at summer camp). This is one reason we haven't missed the removal of fiber from our diet. It consists of strings of glucose molecules such as pectins (found in fruit and used to make jelly) that absorb water to become a gelatinous, viscous substance. Insoluble fiber consists of polysaccharides (non-glucose carbohydrates) such as cellulose, the stringy stuff in celery. They are not digested at all. Because they do not dissolve in water, they have a laxative effect and speed up the passage of food and waste through your gut.

Table 12.1: Sources of Dietary Fiber

Soluble Fiber (absorbs water)	Insoluble Fiber (doesn't absorb water)
oatmeal, oat cereal, lentils, apples, oranges, pears, oat bran, strawberries, nuts, flaxseeds, beans, dried peas, blueberries, psyllium, cucumbers, and carrots	whole wheat, whole grains, wheat bran, corn bran, seeds, nuts, barley, couscous, brown rice, bulgur, zucchini, celery, broccoli, cabbage, onions, tomatoes, celery, carrots, cucumbers, green beans, dark leafy vegetables, fruit, and root vegetable skins

Metabolically, the two together are an unbeatable pair.[3] The insoluble fiber forms a latticework for the soluble fiber to sit on, while the soluble fiber bridges the gaps in the latticework to maintain its integrity—kind of like the hair catcher on your shower drain. Without it, the hair goes down the drain rapidly. But when the hair catcher catches the hair, now you've got a stopped-up bathtub. In the case of fiber, however, inhibiting the rate of flux from the intestine crossing into the bloodstream is a good thing. It gives the liver a chance to fully metabolize what's coming in, so there's no "overflow." Unfortunately, the majority of the foods we are consume today lack fiber of any sort. Refined grains are stripped of both the bran and the germ in the process of milling. This gives them a finer texture and extends their shelf life while taking out various micronutrients (see chapter 14) and, in particular, fiber. Refined grains include white rice, white flour, pasta, potatoes, and many of the cookies, crackers, and cereals that stock your pantry. "Enriched" grains may replace some of the nutrients removed, but once the fiber is taken out you can't put it back in.

The Fallacy Surrounding Fiber

To get the full metabolic benefits of fiber, it needs to "coat" the starch granule on all sides (forming a sphere, or a "kernel") so that the digestive enzymes in the intestine must slowly strip it away. The starch (endosperm) is on the inside. The bran is on the outside. The whole kernel represents a source of insoluble fiber. Strip away the outside bran, and you are left only with the starch (glucose). When you ingest the whole kernel, your intestines will slowly strip away the outside bran, making the rise in serum glucose occur slowly and reach a lower peak concentration. But when the outside bran is removed by processing, your liver is hit with an influx of glucose and the rise occurs quickly, with a higher peak. And that means a higher insulin peak.

So, to derive maximal effects from fiber, you need to consume products with the unadulterated whole grain. Naan and white rice, the only grains in Sujatha's diet, ceased to be grains after being polished at the mill. But here's the problem: even "whole grain" doesn't always mean "whole grain." According to the IOM, food must meet at least one of the following criteria to be considered "whole grain": (1) contain at least 8 grams of whole grain per serving, (2) qualify for the FDA whole grain health claim (51 percent whole grain by weight), or (3) have a whole grain as the first ingredient by weight for non-mixed dishes (e.g., breads, cereals) or as the first grain ingredient by weight for mixed dishes (e.g., pizza, corn dogs). (So "whole grain" Lucky Charms is a misnomer as there are no "whole" grains in the cereal.) Manufacturers may mix in regular starch with the whole grain, but that's not a great idea if you're trying to keep insulin down.

There is nothing in the IOM's definition about the grain being "whole"—that is, uncracked, uncrushed, unadulterated. Plus, foods that list "whole grains" as the second or third ingredient may contain as little as 1 percent. Hence, the IOM definition leaves much to be desired.

The Jive on Juice

Whereas fruit does contain fructose, it also has inherent fiber. And that's not by accident. The reason the fructose in fruit doesn't cause significant health problems is that it's balanced by the endogenous fiber that makes up the solid part of the fruit. If you consume both together, as Nature intended, it reduces the rate of flux to the liver; the liver can keep up, which mitigates most of the negative effects of the sugar. In fact, the amount of fructose in most fruits is balanced nicely by the fruit's fiber content. Conversely, juice is devoid of the insoluble fiber found in whole vegetables and fruits. When "juicing," you keep some of the essential vitamins and minerals (but not all) inherent in the fruit or vegetable, but you discard perhaps the most important part: the fiber. Remember, it doesn't matter where the fructose comes from—fruit, sugarcane, beets—without the fiber, it has the same metabolic effect on your body. Our ancestors didn't have the health complications associated with fructose because they ate the whole fruit.

One current fad is to juice the entire fruit into a "smoothie." Juice bars have popped up all over the West Coast, ostensibly because juicing is healthy. The problem is that the shearing action of the blender blades completely destroys the insoluble fiber of the fruit. The cellulose is torn to smithereens. While the soluble fiber is still there, and can help move food through the intestine faster, it now does not have the "latticework" of the insoluble fiber to help form that intestinal barrier. The sugar in the fruit will be absorbed just as fast as if the juice were strained with no fiber at all. You need both types of fiber to derive the beneficial effects.

Chapter 4 showed us that insulin is the bad guy in terms of weight gain and that keeping insulin down is a priority to combat obesity. The amount and rapidity at which energy arrives at the mitochondria trigger the disease associated with metabolic syndrome (see chapter 9). In other words, the two elements to keep in mind are: the dose of carbohydrate (to keep the insulin down) and the flux of carbohydrates (to keep the liver happy and functioning properly). Fiber takes care of both.

A Waste Product, or a "Waist" Product

As you saw in chapter 11, the glucose in sugar drives the insulin up, while the fructose brings a huge dose of energy straight to the liver for immediate processing, both of which drive obesity and metabolic syndrome (one of the reasons Sujatha developed diabetes). Fiber possesses five different properties that assist in fighting obesity and metabolic syndrome by keeping insulin down and reducing the energy hitting the liver.

1. The Annals of Absorption

Once fiber (soluble and insoluble) is consumed with a meal, it forms a gelatinous barrier between the food and the intestinal wall. This delays the intestine's ability to absorb glucose, fructose, and fat. By slowing glucose absorption, the blood glucose rise is attenuated, which limits the peak glucose. In return, the pancreas, sensing the slower and lower rise in blood glucose, limits its response and reduces the amount of insulin released. Less insulin means less shunting of energy to fat. When patients with type 2 diabetes ate a high-fiber diet, blood sugar was cut by one third, thereby reducing the total insulin load of the body.[4]

The same thing happens with the absorption of fructose.[5] Not only does fiber reduce the dose, it reduces the "flux"—that is, the rate at which fructose is absorbed and arrives at the liver cell for processing. The liver then has a chance to "catch up" and is able to process the fructose molecules to acetyl-CoA at essentially the same rate that new ones are being introduced. This allows them to burn in the mitochondrial Krebs cycle (see chapter 10), instead of overwhelming the mitochondria, to be shunted out and turned into fat, causing subsequent insulin resistance. So, consuming fruit, despite its fructose content, is not nearly as big a problem because the fructose is for the most part mitigated by the presence of fiber.

2. Calories and Cholesterol

Lower blood cholesterol levels are associated with lower rates of heart disease in large populations. One purpose of cholesterol is to aid in the production of bile acids (which help absorb fats in the intestine), some of which are excreted in your stool. So, if you manage to get rid of the bile acids, you lower your cholesterol. Because soluble fiber binds to bile acids, it can help lower LDL ("bad cholesterol"). Insoluble fiber also decreases cholesterol and helps lower blood glucose.

3. Speed and Satiety

You eat a whole plate of macaroni and cheese, yet you're still hungry. Why? Food in the stomach reduces ghrelin levels, which should tell the hypothalamus that you're not hungry anymore. But you still are. The reason is that lack of hunger isn't the same phenomenon as satiety. After food moves through the small intestine, a hormone called peptide $YY_{(3-36)}$ (PYY) is released into the bloodstream, which binds to receptors in the hypothalamus and tells you that you're full. PYY is the satiety signal.[6] The problem is that there are twenty-two feet of intestine that the food has to traverse before the PYY signal is generated. That takes time. So anything that will move the food through the intestine faster will generate the satiety signal sooner. Insoluble fiber does just that; it increases the speed of transit through your gut in order to generate the PYY signal earlier. Soluble fiber forms a sticky gel, delaying the emptying of your stomach, making you feel full faster. Both types of fiber can cut down on the need for consuming second portions, helping to prevent further weight gain.[7]

4. Fat or Fart

With the presence of fiber, some of the dietary fat will be delayed from absorption in the small intestine. Instead, these fiber-delayed dietary fats will make it all the way to the colon, where they won't be absorbed, thus keeping insulin low.[8] Although controversy remains, it is thought that insoluble fiber contributes more significantly to the effects on obesity and insulin resistance than does soluble fiber. The downside of this process is that this fiber will generate a lot of nitrogen, carbon dioxide, methane, and a little hydrogen sulfide in the process. In other words, it's *fat* or *fart*.

5. Bowels and Bugs

The human body contains about ten trillion cells. But your gut harbors about a hundred trillion bacteria. They outnumber us ten to one! For years, we thought they were just along for the ride, making gas at inopportune times and visiting upon us the occasional "traveler's revenge." But those bacteria are a big part of our energy metabolism. Most of the gut bacteria live in the large intestine and are anaerobic, which means they metabolize without oxygen and therefore waste more energy than oxygen burners. Well, if all our nutrients (including fat, glucose, and fructose) are absorbed in our small intestine, what do the large intestinal bacteria have left to eat? What we can't absorb—the fiber, and in particular, the soluble fiber. This is why so many fiber supplements, such as psyllium, give people so much gas.

There are thousands of species of gut bacteria, but science has thus far focused on three: *Bacteroidetes*, *Firmicutes*, and *Archae*. Almost assuredly, the bacterial composition of the gut is one of the factors that promote weight gain in some people. And the fiber composition of the diet is one of the factors that determine the bacterial profile,[9] because fiber delivers more nutrients farther down the intestine, where the bacteria can utilize them for energy.[10] Taken all together, it would appear that altering the fiber content of the diet alters the bacterial content in the gut, allowing for "beneficial" bacteria to proliferate while keeping the "obesogenic" bacteria at bay.[11]

Fiber and Insulin Resistance

So does dietary fiber consumption promote weight loss? Here's where the design of the study makes a big difference. If you keep calorie intake constant, the addition of fiber does not demonstrate significant effects on weight. However, in a free-range situation, where people get to choose how much they eat, higher dietary fiber appears to limit total food intake, which likely results in decreased weight. High-fiber foods tend to be less "energy dense," so you are consuming fewer calories for the same quantity of food. Also they often require more time to chew, giving your body more time to receive its satiety signal, and they move the food through the intestine faster, generating the satiety signal sooner.

The role of dietary fiber in the prevention of metabolic diseases is complicated by which kind of fiber you are talking about and what kind of study you are referring to. In the Insulin Resistance and Atherosclerosis Study (IRAS), dietary analysis demonstrated only one item that correlated with insulin sensitivity: fiber.[12] Yet the soluble fiber content did not corre-late with improvement in diabetes risk.[13] For the most part, this improve-ment in insulin sensitivity was conferred by insoluble fiber (the stringy stuff).[14] So there goes taking soluble fiber supplements such as psyllium. It looks like you have to get your fiber in the food itself, not from a pill. And there's only one way to get both soluble and insoluble fiber: the source—and the closer it is to its original form, the better. This concept of food being better than its components will come up again in chapter 14.

What Comes Out Is Just as Important as What Goes In

It's very clear that fiber is a big deal. Not just for your bowels, but also for your metabolism. Fiber doesn't get absorbed. There's no blood level of fiber, as opposed to levels of micronutrients that improve your metabolic machinery. But by reducing both the dose and the rate of flux of glucose, fructose, and fatty acids entering your bloodstream, fiber keeps your insulin down. By delivering nutrients to the large intestine to allow for fermentation, fiber improves metabolic machinery and selects for the "good" bacteria, which help with energy loss from the colon. Finally, fiber limits total food consumption. But it has to be eaten in the form of the whole, intact food in order to get the full benefit, so you get both the soluble and insoluble fiber. Fiber alone won't mitigate all the negative effects of sugar, but it's a hell of a good start. Want to reverse your diabetes? Want to improve your metabolic health? Put fiber back on the menu.

Chapter 13

Exercise—The Other Half of the Antidote

———————•———————

Britt is a depressed thirteen-year-old boy who weighs 230 pounds and is getting bad grades, in part due to excessive "screen time." His fifteen-year-old brother is 320 pounds and has no intention of altering his lifestyle. Britt sees the misery of his brother and uses him as a "negative role model." Over the next three years, as puberty progresses, Britt starts wrestling in high school, practicing three to four hours a day. He slims down without appreciably altering his diet and without shedding any pounds. He grows into his weight and places second in the state for his weight class. By age eighteen, his depression has lifted, his academics have improved, and he is valedictorian of his high school class.

Jack LaLanne passed away in January 2011 at the ripe old age of ninety-six. The "father" of modern exercise, he adopted a healthy lifestyle at age fifteen and practiced what he preached until the day before his death. He had it right: exercise is the key to optimal health. But not everyone benefits equally. Jim Fixx, one of the pioneer American runners and the author of *The Complete Book of Running*, bit the bullet at age fifty-two. Maybe Fixx died for his first thirty-five years of bad lifestyle choices: before he took up running he smoked two packs per day and weighed 240 pounds. How about Arthur Ashe? The premier tennis player had a heart attack at age thirty-six. Maybe exercise can't reverse a lifetime of indiscretion. Maybe genetic factors play a role. Or maybe exercise has different benefits in different people.

Either way, expecting that exercise will let you live longer is very different from expecting that exercise can help you lose weight. LaLanne didn't gain a pound all those years on TV. That was because he ate properly. Don't get me wrong; there's nothing bad about exercise (although it may not provide all the effects you expect). Exercise is the single best thing you can do for yourself. It's way more important than dieting, and easier to do. Exercise works at so many levels—except one: your weight.

The Myth of Exercise

If "*a calorie is a calorie*" and one ingested equals one burned, then exercise should cause weight loss, and doing a lot of exercise, even if you keep eating the same foods, should make you shed some serious poundage. But it doesn't. The calories you eat or drink may have a positive effect on your weight, but the energy you burn doesn't do the opposite. There is not one study that demonstrates that exercise alone causes significant weight loss, and a meta-analysis (designed to assess significance over many studies at once) proved it; moderate exercise resulted in a weight loss of 2.2 pounds and vigorous exercise in a loss of 3.5 pounds.[1] Given our current obesity epidemic, that just ain't gonna cut it. As an example, a friend of mine decided to clear her post-baby "muffin top" by initiating a moderate-to-vigorous exercise program. Twelve weeks later, she was up five pounds. She felt better, but her muffin top hadn't changed. She asked me what she was doing wrong. Nothing, I told her. She was doing just fine and was likely much healthier than at the outset. Her waist would be smaller, but the muffin top was subcutaneous fat; she could still "pinch the inch." She got into her pre-pregnancy jeans anyway.

Burning a pound of fat liberates 2,500 calories, so it had always been assumed that you can lose one pound by eating 2,500 calories less or exercising 2,500 calories more. However, a recent scientific analysis[2] shows the fallacy of expecting increased energy expenditure to promote weight loss. As people lost weight, their energy intake had to drop even further to keep the weight loss going. On average, obese people had to eat 3,977 calories less to burn off that one pound of fat. So you can see that trying to burn weight off with exercise is extremely difficult, if not downright impossible. A second reason that exercise doesn't cause weight loss is that when you exercise, you build muscle. That's good for your health, but it doesn't reduce your weight.

If chapters 4–9 say anything, it's that studying an event as complex as obesity means looking at the entire gamut of behaviors—because, in the real world, none of them occur in isolation, and all of them are driven by biochemistry. Guaranteed, if you hold food intake constant and then institute vigorous activity, *some* weight loss will follow, but not much. That's why every exercise plan promotes good nutrition. And that's why so many weight-loss programs want to sell you their food. But it's the biochemistry that drives the behavior.

Oh, you say to me, I know people who joined the armed forces and they lost a lot of weight. Wrestlers do it all the time. NFL linemen show up in training camp overweight and out of shape and by the end of exhibition season they're back at playing weight. This is the fact that perpetuates the myth. Anyone can lose weight if his or her *environment* is changed. "Boot camp" is a secluded and controlled environment. Every aspect of your daily regimen, from food to exercise to sleep, is regulated. The trick is to change behavior while in your routine environment. Don't bet the ranch. As we learned in chapter 4, behavior is a result of biochemistry, and biochemistry is a result of environment. Even the contestants on *The Biggest Loser* get a personal trainer and a chef to control their environment. But in a free-range situation, in which the general populace finds itself, energy intake will rise to meet energy expenditure to maintain the same level of adiposity. And in the majority of obese people, we know why: leptin . . . again.

Energy Expenditure in a Nutshell

To explain energy expenditure, we're going to assume a 2,000-calorie intake and 2,000-calorie output for an average person. This value comes both from observation and from the Harris-Benedict equation, a guesstimate used by dietitians to generate dietary plans for individual patients.

Everyone equates energy expenditure with exercise. Your aerobics instructor will yell at you, "Feel the burn." Burning it means *burning* it. In point of fact, physical activity is the minority of energy expenditure, accounting for anywhere from 5 percent (the ultimate couch potato, at about 100 calories) to 35 percent (the gym rat, at about 700 calories) of total energy expenditure based on the level and degree of activity. While physical activity may not account for the largest percentage of energy expenditure, it is the only component that will improve your health—and the more you do, the better.

There are two other components. It might seem hard to believe, but the largest percentage of your calories is burned while sleeping and watching TV (but this does not mean that you should increase your hours on Facebook or World of Warcraft). Resting energy expenditure (REE, the energy you burn lying on the couch) accounts for about 60 percent (or 1,200 calories per day) of total energy expenditure, is dependent on your size, and is usually excluded from concern. Lastly, a process called the thermic effect of food (TEF, the energy you burn to absorb, digest, and metabolize the food you eat) accounts for about 10 percent (or 200 calories). While it's true that for the most part REE and TEF are not easy to change in most people, it should be noted that some patients with obesity exhibit problems with each. And there are some tricks to increase REE and, to a lesser extent, TEF (see chapter 18).

Resting Energy Expenditure

Rudy Leibel at Columbia University in 2004 was quoted as saying, "Obese people tell me all the time they eat very little, they eat like a bird . . . well, maybe a pterodactyl." Yet Rudy himself showed that in response to weight loss, REE declines commensurate with the number of pounds lost, working to keep your weight stable.[3] Don't blame your exercise regimen; blame your biochemistry. While you're burning more energy by going to that Zumba class, your REE is going to thwart you by evening out your overall percentage. Fat cells want to remain filled; they aren't going away without a fight. In response to a decline in either leptin synthesis or leptin signaling (which the hypothalamus interprets as starvation), REE is reduced from 50 calories per kilogram fat-free mass to 42 calories per kilogram fat-free mass, or an improvement in energy efficiency of 16 percent, resulting in a decrease of total energy expenditure of 0.16 x 0.65, or 10 percent. Assuming that standard adult 2,000-calorie intake, that's a decrease of 200 calories, which easily rivals the increase in caloric intake that has been observed in the past thirty years.

Furthermore, there are patients that have specific reductions in REE as part of their general pathology. As REE accounts for the majority of energy expenditure, this is the greatest predictor of weight gain. Children with certain forms of developmental delay are born with lack of muscle tone (called hypotonia) and are "floppy" at birth. Children with various forms of mitochondrial dysfunction (e.g., Prader-Willi syndrome)[4] burn energy at rest about 60–70 percent of normal. This means they need fewer calories. But that means a lower leptin, and their brain feels starved, jacking up the caloric intake.

Thermic Effect of Food (TEF)

You have to put energy in to get energy out. Chewing, moving food through the GI tract, absorbing, and processing food will burn some energy. TEF usually accounts for 10 percent (or 200 calories per day) of all energy burned. Many obese children are not hungry when they awaken (in part because many of them had a big snack or meal just before bedtime), so their body's degree of energy burning is not ratcheted up prior to their departure for school. This is one reason, among many, that eating breakfast is important for prevention and treatment of obesity, especially in children (see chapter 18). Not eating breakfast has many other disadvantages. It means not performing well on tasks because of distraction due to lack of food. Not eating breakfast means the stomach hormone ghrelin, which conveys the signal for hunger, is not suppressed throughout the morning. Obese people rationalize not eating breakfast by saying that's one less meal's worth of calories. That couldn't be further from the truth. Numerous studies show that people who skip breakfast eat *more* during the daylight hours, in part because ghrelin rises to high levels. This leads to overconsumption of calories at lunch, dinner, and prior to bedtime, all driving further obesity.

Even though oxidation of fats (see chapter 10) liberates a lot of energy, a little bit of energy is spent making it work. Another way to take advantage of TEF to is to consume some form of protein at breakfast. Burning protein costs more energy than burning other foodstuffs.[5] Protein does not stimulate insulin to the same extent as carbohydrates do, and increases satiety better than other nutrients. So consuming some protein at breakfast is a smart and very defensible practice. People who eat veggie omelets at breakfast are way less hungry at lunchtime.[6]

Physical Activity

Finally, physical activity. You can be completely sedentary, or you can be Olympic swimmer Michael Phelps. The range of energy expenditure by physical activity that humans can achieve is quite remarkable; topped perhaps only by how many calories can be eaten. Phelps eats everything in sight, on the order of 12,000 calories a day. As hard as he works, he doesn't expend 12,000 calories in physical activity—even marathon runners don't burn that kind of energy. The Cleveland Clinic Center for Consumer Health estimates that a 130-pound runner will burn 2,224 calories during a marathon, a 165-pound runner will burn 2,822 calories, and a 210-pound runner will burn 3,593 calories. Yet Phelps can eat anything he wants, and he doesn't gain weight. That's because exercise increases the number of mitochondria in the form of increased muscle. And increased muscle means you burn more energy at rest. So Michael Phelps has a higher REE than you do. And that's why exercise is good; because it builds muscle, and muscle burns energy even at rest.

Physical activity is the most misunderstood aspect of obesity medicine. People think if they exercise they will lose weight. That's a pipe dream. Most of the studies of exercise for obesity in children are free-range community interventions and use either weight or BMI as their outcome. And no amount of exercise is going to change BMI, a measure of body size, because BMI is the wrong outcome. In the absence of environmental control, caloric intake will increase to meet the shortfall. Remember, your subcutaneous fat can actually be good for you. But as discussed in chapter 8, the target of exercise is muscle and bone.

What Exercise Actually Does

So, if you're not going to lose weight, why go to spin class? Why is exercise so good for you? Diet is about pounds, exercise is about inches. Diet is about weight, exercise is about health. Exercise does the one thing that dietary restriction cannot: it builds muscle. This is a poorly understood concept, because most people, including clinicians, equate BMI with body fat. BMI does not take into account the difference between muscle and fat, or the difference between subcutaneous and visceral fat. Several studies have examined body composition before and after long-term exercise. What they show is that percentage body fat declined. Absolutely true. But it's because muscle increased. And, in the process, metabolic status improved— both because visceral fat went down (a little) and because muscle went up (a lot) (see chapter 8).

You *want* to improve your insulin sensitivity—and exercise does just that. It makes you build muscle at the expense of visceral and especially liver fat. But you can't see this by stepping on a scale. By improving insulin sensitivity and lowering insulin levels, exercise improves leptin signaling, thereby increasing your sympathetic tone (see chapter 4), energy expenditure, and quality of life.

And these metabolic improvements translate into disease prevention. A study of thirty-eight thousand American men showed that physical activity was more potent in preventing heart disease than being normal weight.[7] But what about the ultimate outcome: does exercise promote longevity? A recent study out of Taiwan looking at the death rates of over four hundred thousand subjects suggests that moderate-intensity exercise for fifteen minutes a day could increase lifespan by as much as three years, even in patients with known heart disease.[8] And they didn't control for diet; if they had, they would have seen an even greater effect of exercise on longevity. Given that 15 minutes a day accounts for only 91 waking hours a year, or 273 hours in 3 years, a 3-year life extension for 273 hours of exercise performed is a pretty darn good trade.

The Biochemistry of Exercise

Exercise is truly the other half of the antidote. It will not cure obesity, but it goes a long way toward mitigating all its negative effects, especially those of metabolic syndrome (see chapter 9). Biochemically, exercise does three things:

1. Exercise directly activates your sympathetic nervous system (SNS) (see chapter 4). The SNS sends a signal to your muscles to make new mitochondria, which means that more energy (glucose or fatty acids) can be burned. The age of mitochondria plays a big role, because old mitochondria are inefficient, "leaky," and make more ROS (see chapter 9), which contributes to insulin resistance. Exercise clears away those old mitochondria, allowing for clean, efficient use of energy by muscles.[9] This improves muscle insulin sensitivity, which is key to improving your general metabolic health.

2. Exercise is your internal stress reducer. Britt became a well-adjusted teenager (not always an oxymoron) in part because he started to work out. While blood cortisol levels (see chapter 6) rise immediately upon exercise (as they are part of the process that keeps your blood sugar and blood pressure up), they come down quickly, and stay down the rest of the day.[10] To reduce your blood pressure, you may want to consider exercise—not because your weight will go down, but because exercising will reduce your stress levels and release endorphins (feel-good chemicals in your brain) to make you feel better throughout the day. This is how runners get their "runner's high." We want to keep our cortisol levels low to improve our long-term metabolic status. A little pain, a lot of gain.

3. Perhaps most important, exercise increases the speed of your liver's Krebs cycle (see chapters 9 and 11) and makes it burn energy cleaner.[11] This determines how much energy will be shuttled out of the mitochondria and converted to liver fat. Four factors have been shown to speed up the liver's Krebs cycle: cold, altitude, the thyroid hormone (we gave extra thyroid hor-

mone to obese women back in the 1960s and it made them crazy), and exercise. Cold and altitude are a potent anti-obesity combination. Take the difference between Switzerland and Germany. Switzerland eats virtually the same diet as does Germany. Fat and carbohydrate together, an obesogenic diet if I ever saw one. Lots of potatoes, lots of bread, lots of cheese, lots of cream sauces, lots of beer. Yum. Their rates of physical activity are also virtually the same. But Switzerland is high, cold, and thin (only 8 percent obesity), while Germany is low, less cold, and fat (16 percent obesity). Same thing in Colorado: you're so proud because the CDC obesity map shows that you're the least obese state in the United States. But I know the real reason you've lagged behind the rest of the country, and it isn't your food or your active lifestyle—it's your geography. So, everyone, if you don't want to exercise, move to Switzerland or Colorado!

Cardio or Isometric Exercise?

Assuming you're a mere mortal at sea level and not an Olympian on a mountain, what kind of exercise should you perform to get the health benefits? The standard mantra was that low-intensity, long-interval exercise, otherwise known as "cardio" (e.g., running), worked your heart and provided all the cardiovascular benefits. There were even those who eschewed resistance or isometric exercise because it temporarily reduced the blood flow to the heart, thus slowing it, and because it increased peripheral muscle, it did not promote weight loss. But recent prospective studies show that high-intensity interval training (fits of extreme activity interspersed with low levels of exercise)[12] or even strength training (weight lifting)[13] provide equal improvements in waist circumference and blood vessel flow. So, don't sweat what kind of exercise, just sweat!

It's All Good, Except When It's Not

Of course, you can overdo exercise. Exercise promotes the release of chemicals called "endogenous opioids," or "endorphins," which cause the hypothalamus to reduce the release of the pituitary hormones luteinizing hormone (LH) and follicle-stimulating hormone (FSH), which reduces estrogen production by the ovaries. In women, this leads to the stoppage of menses and long-term reductions in bone mass—not a good thing, given that women are destined to lose bone mass rapidly upon menopause.

When obese patients start to exercise, they may be at significant risk for injury because of the excess weight they are carrying. The obese need to exercise to improve their overall health, but they need to start out slowly, because they are at greater risk for muscle strains and pulls as well as fractures. Studies demonstrate that the fracture rate among the obese is four times higher than the general population.[14]

And the biggest problem of all: the beneficial effects of exercise, while excellent for your body and your metabolism, are relatively short-lived, and have to be frequent and sustained. Studies demonstrate that levels of PPAR-gamma coactivator 1-alpha (PGC-1α; the protein in muscle cells that turns on all the good muscle metabolic effects and tells the mitochondria to divide) decline within a day of cessation of exercise, and insulin sensitivity returns to baseline within fifteen days.[15] So, those of you weekend warriors who think you're doing yourself some good—it may not be as good as you think. If you're going to use exercise as your protection against chronic disease, you'll have to be consistent about it.

Fat and Fit Is Better Than Thin and Sick

Exercise is the other half of the antidote. It is your best defense against metabolic dysfunction. Here's another way to look at it. Every molecule of energy that you absorb has one of three fates: First, you can burn it, in which case your insulin doesn't rise, you won't gain weight, and you won't do metabolic damage. Second, you can store it, in which case your insulin goes up, you gain weight, and you do some metabolic damage. Or third, the energy goes out in your urine, in which case you wreak complete metabolic havoc and cause kidney damage, as seen in poorly controlled diabetics who end up on dialysis. Burning energy is always preferable to the other two options. Just don't expect exercise to induce weight loss, unless it is coupled with some sort of dietary intervention as well.

So let's go back to chapters 1 and 9, where I mentioned that 40 percent of normal-weight individuals are insulin resistant or have metabolic syndrome, and those who do also have fatty livers. Who do you think is better off? The fat person who exercises, or the thin one who watches nonstop *Law & Order* marathons? Recent studies have demonstrated that fitness mitigates all the negative effects of obesity on visceral fat,[16] health complaints,[17] and longevity.[18] So does the fat and fit person deserve to be discriminated against? As long as she keeps it up, she'll likely live longer than the stick thin model on the cover of *Vogue*. Indeed, overweight people with BMIs between 25 and 30 live longer than thin people with BMIs of less than 19.[19]

The Greatest Disservice, and by the Medical Profession

Nonetheless, doctors continue to promote the party line with their obese patients. The corollary to "*a calorie is a calorie*" is the mantra "If you'd only exercise, you'd lose weight." Not only is this wrong, it's downright detrimental. Patients who monitor their exercise progress on a home scale are destined for disappointment. But their doctors tell them it will work, and the patients trust them. So they think they're failures, get depressed, and stop exercising and start eating, because they think it's no use. A great way to make metabolic syndrome even worse. Irrespective of weight, consistent exercise (even just fifteen minutes a day) is the single best way for people to improve their health. That's 273 hours paid in for 3 years of life gained, or a 64,000 percent return on investment. The best deal in all of medicine.

Chapter 14

Micronutrients: Home Run or Hyperbole?

————————•————————

Julio is a fifteen-year-old Latino male from West Texas who weighs 400 pounds. He is Med-Flighted to San Francisco for an emergency liver transplant because his pathology shows severe fatty liver and scarring, known as nonalcoholic steatohepatitis (NASH) with cirrhosis, a condition associated with severe alcohol abuse. Although he has never consumed alcohol, he has imbibed at least a half-gallon of Coca-Cola every day since he was old enough to open the refrigerator. Julio's transplant is successful, and he is discharged two weeks later, after being told to lose weight, stop drinking soda, and improve his diet. One year later, Julio is seen back at UCSF for a checkup. His diet hasn't changed, the soft drinks continue, his weight has not declined, and an ultrasound shows fatty deposits in his new liver.

No doubt Julio's new liver will suffer the same fate. Nonalcoholic fatty liver disease (NAFLD) is now the most common disease in America, affecting 45 percent of all Latinos, 33 percent of all Caucasians, and 24 percent of all African Americans, fat and thin. Considering this disease was not even described until 1980, the increase in prevalence to encompass one third of the entire adult population is astounding. Most of the people with NAFLD have no symptoms and don't even know they have it. The majority of them will suffer no ill effects. But 5 percent of them will go on to develop NASH, with inflammation and scarring of the liver. And of those, 25 percent will develop cirrhosis, which will lead either to death or to a liver transplant, just as with Julio. When you do the math, that's one million Americans dying from a nutritional disease; never mind all those who die from other complications of metabolic syndrome. Considering that this disease is completely preventable, this is a travesty. But is this an *overnutritional* disease or an *undernutritional* disease? Both, as it turns out.

While there are certain genetic predispositions (accounting for the higher prevalence in Latinos), you still need the excess energy coursing through the liver to develop the disease. Cue the sugar glut. We aren't certain why the disease affects some severely, while remaining benign in others. There are several theories. Remember our biological enemies, the reactive oxygen species (ROS; see chapter 9)? Those whose livers can't quench (detoxify) their ROS will progress on to NASH. ROSs damage lipids and proteins within the cell, which can cause cell structural damage or cell death. Removal of ROSs before they can do damage is the job of a subcellular structure called the peroxisome, which is where ROSs go to die. The chemicals that do the dirty work of knocking them off are known as antioxidants.

The "Triage Hypothesis"

It's been over a hundred years since we discovered the link between vitamin B_1 and beriberi, a disease of cardiac and neurological degeneration. William Fletcher discovered that eating polished rice stripped of its fiber caused the disease, while eating unpolished rice prevented it. Since then, we've learned of many vitamin or mineral deficiencies that lead to specific individual diseases with funny names (e.g., scurvy, pellagra). Fortunately, virtually all these micronutrient deficiency diseases have been essentially wiped out in America—either through the abundance of micronutrients in our diet or through specific supplementation in foods (such as giving folic acid to pregnant women to prevent neural tube defects in newborns). The concept that the diseases of metabolic syndrome might be due to inadequate micronutrient availability has been spurred on by animal studies and small-scale human studies. Nonetheless, the search for the "magic supplement" to reverse metabolic syndrome continues with fervor.

Enter Bruce Ames at Children's Hospital Oakland Research Institute, who has been working in the field of nutrition for fifty years. He has put forward the "triage hypothesis" to explain our current metabolic dilemma. The premise is simple: Cells want to survive. Virtually every biochemical reaction requires one micronutrient or other, whether it is a vitamin, mineral, or biochemical compound. When micronutrients are in short supply, they are triaged to these reactions to maintain cell viability. Their relative deficiency then deprives secondary reactions, which are less important to short-term survival but crucial for long-term cell integrity. DNA or protein damage that goes unrepaired can lead to either cancer formation or cell death. According to the triage hypothesis, acute micronutrient deficiency leads to one set of diseases (e.g., scurvy), while relative micronutrient insufficiency leads to another set of diseases (e.g., metabolic syndrome).

I Used to Care, but Now I Take a Pill for That . . .

As our collective health has declined over the past thirty years, the imperative to find the magic bullet that will forgive our previous indiscretions has only heightened. This has created the approximately $100 billion industry of "nutraceuticals." Currently, more than 50 percent of America takes at least one form of nutritional supplement, hedging their bets. A trip to the local health food store or pharmacy will overwhelm even the most seasoned vitamin aficionado with options. Do any of these supplements exert any benefits? Maybe it doesn't matter, since 71 percent of users say their belief is so strong that they will continue to consume the nutraceutical even if studies demonstrate a lack of efficacy.

Antioxidants: The Fountains of Youth?

Almost every advertisement for breakfast cereal shows the bowl dressed with a handful of blueberries. Perhaps this is to draw your attention away from the fact that the antioxidants in the cereal have been processed out and that the only way to rescue your meal is to supplement them back in the form of fresh berries. No doubt, more color means more antioxidants, and fruits and vegetables are packed with them. Antioxidants allow the plant to buffer the damage from its own ROSs when making its carbohydrates from photosynthesis. Can consuming them help us to battle our own?

There's growing literature that "oxidative stress," or the damage caused by ROSs, is the single most important factor contributing to the aging process. Different tissues generate ROSs by different means. Therefore, disparate antioxidants are required to help quench them to prevent various types of chronic diseases. Antioxidants come in many shapes and sizes, many of which have been considered as treatments for metabolic syndrome.[1] The antioxidants vitamins C and E protect against lipid peroxidation (as in potato chips when they go rancid), though neither has been shown to improve vascular function or insulin resistance. In fact, high-dose vitamin E has been linked to increased rates of mortality.[2] Although there are occasional "hits" among the treatment of metabolic diseases with antioxidants, most are near misses.

Vitamin D—The "Great Impostor"?

By far, the most enticing yet unrealized hope for the magic bullet that will cure all our ills is vitamin D. More has been written about this compound than all other vitamins, minerals, and supplements combined. Deficiency of vitamin D can occur either from lack of sunlight (which makes vitamin D in the skin) or lack of vitamin D in the diet. Vitamin D is certainly a godsend for children who suffer from rickets, a debilitating bone disease and seizure disorder due to a lack of vitamin D. We learned back in the 1920s that a teaspoon of castor oil (made from salmon liver) cured rickets, though we didn't know why (much to the chagrin of the children forced to swallow it). In the 1950s it was discovered that a teaspoon of castor oil contained 400 units of vitamin D, so this became the dogma: we need 400 units of vitamin D per day (although recent studies suggest we need as much as 800 per day).

Could low vitamin D be at the heart of our chronic metabolic problems? Many scientists subscribe to this idea, and a subset of them have gone out on a limb to stake their claim to vitamin D as the cure-all for chronic metabolic disease. There is no doubt that vitamin D levels correlate inversely with all the core diseases associated with metabolic syndrome: diabetes, hypertension, and heart disease. But why is one third of America vitamin D deficient anyway? One reason is that we have been taught to avoid the sun like the plague. The second reason is that per capita consumption of milk, the primary source of dietary vitamin D, has declined by half over the past sixty years. Commensurate with the decline in milk consumption is the increase in sugar-sweetened beverages (soda and juice). You can't untie the two with epidemiologic data, which is all we have so far. So which is the cause of metabolic syndrome? The dearth of vitamin D, the glut of sugar, or a combination of the two? Currently, not one study examines vitamin D levels and sugar consumption at the same time to determine which is the primary cause of metabolic syndrome and which is secondary.[3]

Resveratrol: The New "It" Compound

Perhaps the single biggest blockbuster in the field of nutraceuticals is in trials right now. Not since gingko biloba has a nutraceutical been so highly touted as has resveratrol, a compound found in small amounts in food but in high amounts in red wine. (Yes, you *can* have it all!) But this one has some staying power because of its mechanism of action in the right part of the cell. In animal models, resveratrol has shown beneficial effects on reducing inflammation produced by ROSs and, by doing so, preventing cancer, reducing atherosclerosis, reducing visceral fat, improving insulin sensitivity, and possibly even preserving neuronal function—all with virtually no side effects. The problem is that human studies are just getting started, and so far have been short term only. The most recent review[4] suggests that while promising, resveratrol is not yet ready for prime time.

Contenders or Pretenders?

Many epidemiologic studies demonstrate correlations between low blood levels of antioxidants such as vitamin C and beta-carotene and the prevalence of metabolic syndrome. But are these micronutrient deficiencies the true cause of disease or just markers of an extremely bad diet? At this point, we just don't know. We know that altering *diet* (eating more fruits and vegetables, limiting processed foods and sugar) to deliver more of these compounds is almost uniformly beneficial in improving the signs and symptoms of metabolic syndrome. But when these antioxidants are given as supplements, they usually fail miserably. This could very well be due to the beneficial effects of eating unprocessed foods, where you get both the fiber and the antioxidants as a bonus.

In clinical trials, vitamin E supplementation has flamed out not once but five separate times: (1) in the Alpha-Tocopherol, Beta-Carotene Cancer Prevention (ATBC) study, in which beta-carotene (the orange stuff in carrots and the precursor to vitamin A) and vitamin E given to heavy smokers increased their risk for cancer and ischemic heart disease; (2) in the Heart Outcomes Prevention Education (HOPE) Trial of 2005, in which vitamin E contributed to heart failure; (3) in the Women's Health Initiative of 2005, in which ten years of vitamin E showed no benefit on heart disease or cancer; (4) in the Selenium and Vitamin E Cancer Prevention Trial (SELECT) of 2009, in which the vitamin E group increased their risk for prostate cancer; and (5) in a 2008 Cochrane meta-analysis, in which vitamin E did not alter the rate of cognitive decline.

The Iowa Women's Health Study has provided the most recent stake through the heart for the dietary supplement movement.[5] This long-term and well-controlled study showed slightly *increased* risk of death with several dietary supplements (particularly iron). Of all of them, the only long-term benefit was found by taking calcium, which improved longevity through fewer broken bones. But you never hear about these failures, because no agency publicizes them and there is no pressure to remove the supplements from the market.

This is a real dilemma. Micronutrients matter—the biochemistry says so—except they don't work when provided as supplements in clinical trials. How many studies do we need? Now you're ready for the dénouement: Real food, containing endogenous micronutrients, prevents metabolic syndrome. Processed food causes metabolic syndrome. And nutritional supplements can't reverse that which has previously been destroyed.[6] So why does real food work while supplements don't?

The Right Stuff: Real versus Manufactured

Face it, we got spoiled by previous successes. All the classic vitamins work to cure their respective nutritional deficiencies, even when they are supplied in a pill. Perhaps because the only thing that's wrong is the undernutrition, the vitamin deficiency itself. But metabolic syndrome is far more complicated. Treating overnutrition is a much tougher nut to crack. Replacing something that's missing is a whole lot easier than taking away something that's in excess. Kind of like pudding. You can always put it back on the stove. But once overcooked, you might as well throw it away. There are five theories as to why:

1. Various items added during the processing of food, such as sugar and other preservatives, are even more toxic than we think (see chapter 12). Something that ubiquitous and potent may just dwarf the beneficial effects of any nutritional supplement.
2. The processing of food removes something even more valuable than the micronutrients, which remain un-replaced. Could there be something else in real food that is missing in processed food? Could it be the fiber itself? Could fiber be the real antidote to metabolic syndrome while everything else is just window dressing?
3. The simple act of food processing removes the food's native micronutrients, just as the fiber is stripped. After all, many micronutrients travel with the fiber. Recall the beriberi story—it was the

polished rice, stripped of its fiber, that lost its native vitamin B_1. Flavonoids, folate, and many other micronutrients are decimated by food processing. While it's enticing to think that we can put them back with a pill, the data support that once a food is "biologically" dead, it's unlikely that you can revive it with a sprinkling of a nutraceutical.

4. Some antioxidants when furnished in high supply are instead oxidants, performing the opposite effect. The perfect example of this is iron. Iron is needed to make all the scavenger enzymes work, but too much iron brings its own level of oxidation—it's called rust, which like the "browning reaction," occurs inside you as well.

5. Nutraceutical supplements aren't subject to the same rigorous quality control standards as pharmaceuticals. The Dietary Supplement Health and Education Act of 1994, passed by Congress, virtually assured the nutraceutical industry a free pass on demonstrating both safety and efficacy of their products. In 2008 the IOM crafted lower limits for these substances, but no tolerable upper intake limits—which means that companies don't have to assure potency. Can you assure consistency from one batch to the next? Can you even assure that the native plant was accurately identified and put in the correct supplement? And does consuming 1,000 percent of your USDA recommended daily allowance of vitamin C have any demonstrable effects on fighting the common cold? The only way that the industry has gotten away with this so far is that the FDA doesn't regulate them.

One thing's for sure: the $123.9 billion (in 2008) nutraceutical industry, accounting for 6 percent of all food dollars, is a house of cards. Better to go with the tried-and-true answer to combat metabolic syndrome. We know it works, it has even more positive effects for our bodies, it's a lot cheaper, and it tastes better. So what is this magic bullet? Unfortunately for Julio, it's not a new liver. Rather, it's called *real food*.

Chapter 15

Environmental "Obesogens"

———————•———————

Rebecca is a five-year-old girl who has gained 20 pounds in one year and is referred to us for premature breast development. An MRI of her head rules out a brain tumor. A pituitary evaluation to look for the onset of puberty is unrevealing, and tests show no estrogen in the blood. A more detailed history reveals that Rebecca's mother has recently taken to bathing her daughter in Victoria's Secret bath gel. The bottle says in large block lettering, "FOR ADULTS ONLY." The assumption is that the bath gel contains a plant estrogen. The mother is counseled to stop the bath gel, and subsequently Rebecca's weight gain and breast development both cease.

In 1990 no U.S. state had an obesity rate higher than 14 percent. In just twenty years, not one state is absolved from having a population with a lower obesity rate than 20 percent; thirty-six states have a prevalence of 25 percent or more. These numbers continue to climb, with no signs of abating. Perhaps the most bizarre thing about the obesity pandemic is its spread over time. To think that this national trend is purely a mass alteration in behavioral change, state by state, is to ignore the pattern of this pandemic. Rather, it is more akin to an infectious disease, a contagion, or some other mass environmental exposure. But what can have that effect and that sort of reach?

The Obesity/Puberty Dilemma

One of the issues that directed attention to the childhood obesity epidemic, and the possibility of some grand and overwhelming exposure, is the fact that girls have been starting puberty at increasingly younger ages.[1] Understandably, this is causing parents undue distress. Studies have demonstrated that, across ethnicities, girls are exhibiting breast development as young as seven years of age: Caucasians (10 percent), African Americans (23 percent), and Latinos (15 percent).[2] Many studies have since corroborated the finding of earlier-onset puberty in girls (but not in boys; we don't know why). Coinciding with the epidemic of early breast development in girls is the epidemic of obesity. Could the two be related? Could it be that the breast development (and perhaps also obesity) is not being caused by the ovary (true puberty), but rather some kind of estrogen exposure?

For hundreds of years the timing of puberty in girls has been advancing earlier and earlier. This advancement has been attributed to improved nutrition and increased weight and fat at younger ages. Higher BMI clearly predicts earlier menarche,[3] which suggests that obesity may be the culprit of the recent early-onset puberty. Furthermore, we know that children who constantly exercise vigorously and don't gain weight, such as gymnasts and ballet dancers (many of whom also suffer from eating disorders), won't enter puberty at all until they slow down. In addition, their growth is often stunted. This is a perfect example of how the hormone leptin is a permissive factor in the onset and progression of puberty; you have to gain a certain amount of fat to generate the leptin needed to start the process—no leptin, no puberty.[4]

Due to all this obesity, leptin levels are increasing at younger ages—but is puberty really occurring as early as age seven or not? We're still not sure how to interpret the data because there are two questions that have yet to be answered. First, is the appearance of breast tissue in girls always a true sign of the onset of puberty? Could it just be fat tissue making the breasts look bigger? You would have to palpate (feel) the breast tissue to be sure; and many of these studies used visual inspection only. (Many doctors feel uncomfortable palpating the breasts of young girls.) Second, how do we know that breast development truly means that puberty has begun? This is not always clear because it depends on the source of the estrogen, and we don't always know where the estrogen is coming from.

Three sources of estrogen can promote breast development: First, the ovary—when the hypothalamus gets the leptin signal, it can allow the pubertal process to begin. Second, the fat cells, which have the enzyme that makes estrogen—the more fat, the more estrogen. This is true in both women and men (hence obese men get "man boobs" and sometimes need the "manzierre"). Third, any chemical in the environment that resembles estrogen, which could induce breast tissue formation and fat storage. A chemical that disrupts the endocrine system. An *environmental obesogen*.

What Is an Obesogen?

Scientists have coined the term *obesogen* to refer to any endocrine-disrupting chemical (EDC) that promotes weight gain and obesity in people. Obesogens can promote obesity in various ways. Like estrogen, they can increase the number of, or promote fat storage into, existing fat cells. Obesogens can alter energy balance to favor the storage of calories and reduce the amount of calories burned at rest (REE; see chapter 13). They can change the mechanisms through which the body experiences appetite or satiety. In other words, obesogens can insidiously hijack the body's energy balance system, making energy go places that are detrimental to your metabolic health.

Estrogens

It doesn't take much for any chemical to be an estrogen. The human estrogen receptor is extraordinarily promiscuous; it'll hook up with just about any chemical that strikes its fancy. And there loads of chemicals that make the estrogen receptor go wild and lose all its inhibitions, promoting breast development and inducing fat cell differentiation, which means weight gain as well.

Estrogens are *everywhere*. They are in our food, our plastics, and our water supply. Until recently they were used in our pesticides. Perhaps the most famous of these compounds is the pesticide DDT. Used in great abundance during World War II to control malaria and typhus among the troops, this chemical worked to kill off insects because it was an estrogen. Rachel Carson's 1962 book *Silent Spring* indicated that DDT was a cause of animal disease and human cancer. The pesticide was banned in the United States in 1972 and in Mexico in 1997. Here's the kicker: DDT has been absent from the United States for four decades, yet its metabolite DDE can still be found in the urine of pregnant women, even those who were born *after* 1972. Among the many implications for health, the concentration of DDE in pregnant women's urine predicts the weight of their children at age three.[5] Almost assuredly, DDE is creating extra fat cells before the baby is even born! Could this be driving childhood obesity?

Another well-known estrogen is our newest environmental bogeyman, bisphenol-A, or BPA. This compound is leeched out every time an acid touches a polycarbonate plastic bottle. In other words, every consumable liquid in America. BPA is used in a multitude of commercial products. The BPA-cancer link is strong enough that the state of California has passed a ban of BPA in baby bottles and kids' toys that will go into effect in 2013. BPA is associated with fat cell differentiation, and urine BPA concentrations are correlated with BMI in adults.[6] But remember, correlation is *not* causation.

The last of our big-time estrogen exposures is genistein, a soy and alfalfa estrogen. Genistein drives fat cell differentiation in rats; exposure at birth predicts increased fat deposition at three and four months. And because it's in soy, it's in everything we eat. Even if you're a carnivore, the meat you consume will be from animals that were fed soy products. If you are a vegetarian, you'll still be ingesting it in your milk and cheese. And vegans are likely eating lots of soy products anyway (e.g., tofu), so no one is immune. Whether genistein contributes to human obesity is still unknown, and the data are being collected now. However, given the ubiquity of soy products in our food supply, it's still a cause for concern.

Phthalates

Like that new shower curtain smell? Those are phthalates, plasticizers that render plastics soft and pliable. Phthalates are used in a large variety of items, from the coatings on pharmaceutical pills and nutritional supplements to personal care products, to children's products such as rubber duckies. In adults, urine phthalate levels correlate with adiposity, waist circumference, and insulin resistance. And most recently, phthalate levels in the urine correlated with waist circumference in New York City children.[7] Again, while this is correlation and not causation, it is still highly worrisome.

Atrazine and Other Organochlorines

Atrazine is an example of an organochlorine, a pesticide that is highly teratogenic, that is, causing structural malformations in living things (e.g., tadpoles). This has implications for human developmental abnormalities and childhood cancer. Atrazine use has been banned in Europe but not in the United States. Iowa is awash in atrazine because it is the chief pesticide for the state's corn crop. For the past two decades, there has been a "dead zone" in the northern Gulf of Mexico, killing nearly all the fish in the Delta, due to the atrazine runoff down the Mississippi River. Blood atrazine levels correlate with adiposity and insulin resistance in adults. But again, showing that atrazine *causes* human obesity is still a long way off.

Tributyltin (TBT)

Tributyltin, or TBT, is not a well-known compound, but it is particularly egregious when it comes to obesity. TBT is a fungicide, used in painting ships to prevent rotting and keep barnacles from sticking to the hull. Because it's on boats, it's also in our general water supply, meaning that everyone is exposed to it. When it comes to making fat, TBT does double duty.[8] First, it mimics the signals that tell fat cells to multiply; and second, it activates cortisol metabolism so that more visceral fat accumulates (see chapter 6). Bad news all around. Worse yet, a single exposure for a pregnant rat promotes fatty liver in her offspring right at birth, dooming them to a lifetime of obesity and metabolic syndrome. Although we can measure TBT in human urine (so we know we're exposed), the jury is still out as to whether TBT is a primary driver of obesity in either children or adults.

Smoking and Air Pollution

Everyone knows that smoking is bad news. Yet despite Surgeon General Luther Terry declaring that smoking was harmful to health in 1964, it took thirty years for society to care enough to do anything about it. Why has society enacted these changes now? Thanks to the rights of the nonsmoker, we now have no-smoking laws in public buildings. All this because of secondhand smoke. And no one suffers more than the unborn child.

Cigarette smoke harbors a host of ugly compounds, one of which is thiocyanate, a relative of cyanide. Thiocyanate inhibits the function of the thyroid gland and is known to reduce thyroid levels in school-age children whose parents smoke. This might alter cognitive performance in school. Worse yet, thiocyanate crosses the placenta to the fetus and is also found in breast milk. Cigarette smoking is a well-known cause of SGA (small for gestational age) in newborns and, as elaborated on in chapter 7, SGA infants are at high risk for developing obesity and metabolic syndrome in later life.

But the chemicals you breathe in every day could be even more insidious than someone else's smoke. One of the most sobering associations, and one that may play a huge role in the worldwide obesity and diabetes pandemics, is air pollution. There is no question that obesity and diabetes rates have increased progressively in industrialized countries. The counterpart to the "*a calorie is a calorie*" argument is that we now drive everywhere instead of walk, so we don't burn the energy. Another dogma to be shattered. We've long known that asthma, obesity, and diabetes like to congregate in the same individual. Several new studies have shown that living near freeways or other highways is a major risk factor for developing all three. A long-term study of ten-year-olds in Southern California showed that the level of traffic within 150 meters of a child's home predicted that child's BMI by age eighteen.[9] What is not clear is whether the air quality had direct effects, or whether the degree of traffic altered the child's level of physical activity and thus promoted weight gain.

Or Is It an Infection?

This whole book is about the obesity *pandemic*—and a pandemic it is. But when we talk about pandemics, we're usually talking about some contagion such as influenza, plague, ebola, or something equally movie-worthy. The pattern of obesity propagation looks like some grand exposure. Could it be due to some sort of infection?

Enter adenovirus-36 (Ad-36). This virus starts by giving you standard cold symptoms and then takes over your fat cells. Ad-36 does just what some of these EDCs do: it differentiates your fat cells and makes them divide. Standard transmission studies have shown that infection of monkeys with Ad-36 makes them gain weight. And like any other adenovirus (respiratory infections), Ad-36 is contagious through coughing and sneezing. For obvious reasons, proving causation in humans is a little harder to do. However, Ad-36 antibody levels correlate with BMI in certain populations, particularly in children.[10] In one study, 15 percent of obese children were Ad-36-positive, compared to 7 percent of normal-weight children. But *within* the obese population, those who were Ad-36-positive weighed, on average, 35 pounds more than those who were not. This suggests that Ad-36 might make the obese get obeser. But all these correlations are still not causation. We have a long way to go before we can prove that Ad-36 is a bona fide contributor to human obesity.

You Can Run, but You Can't Hide

I could go on—the list of offending agents seems endless. And of course, let's not forget the most ubiquitous toxin of them all: fructose, the Evil Queen/Witch of this story, peddling the poison we just can't get enough of.

No one can escape. These EDCs are everywhere. We've got toxins in the water, plastics, grocery store, and in the very air we breathe. Rebecca may have been affected by obesogens in her bath gel. Indeed, even animal species that drink our water, breathe our air, and eat chow made from the same adulterated foodstuffs (corn, soy) are also getting fatter[11] (see chapter 3).

You still don't want to try to argue that obesity is due to gluttony and sloth, do you?

The obesogen hypothesis makes two important points. First, susceptibility to obesity is part of the human (and animal) condition. These chemicals *love* to make fat cells, and fat cells *love* to get filled. Second, obesogens can alter developmental programming of fat cells or the hypothalamus *in utero*, and thus change the set point for gaining weight as early as birth. Even though the exposure might end, the damage appears to last forever. And there are more of them around today than ever before.

Finally, back to our obese six-month-old. Soy infant formulas are packed with these compounds, and consuming soy formula is a well-known contributor to weight gain. The formula Isomil is 10.3 percent sucrose (Coca-Cola is 10.5 percent sucrose). It's a baby milkshake! Add to that the genistein in the soy formula, and put all that in a baby bottle containing bisphenol-A. Is that six-month-old looking more like a perpetrator or victim?

How can we reduce our exposure to EDCs? Sadly, reducing such environmental exposure usually requires governmental legislation and public health intervention. Does any government agency have the stomach for that? We'll address the public health implications of the obesity pandemic in part 6.

Chapter 16

The "Empire" Strikes Back: Response of the Food Industry

———————•———————

"Obesity is a complex problem with many causes and no single, easy solution. It is irresponsible and scientifically spurious to single out HFCS or any other food or ingredient as the chief cause of obesity. The only effective and lasting way to combat obesity is to encourage people to live a balanced lifestyle, eating a variety of foods in moderation and incorporating lots of physical activity into their daily lives."

—National Soft Drink Association press release, March 25, 2004

Sort of. HFCS and sucrose are, for all intents and purposes, biochemically and metabolically equivalent. But the truth stops there. Both the Sugar Association and the Corn Refiners Association have gone out of their way in their attempts to exonerate sugar, whatever the source. They want the public to think that *"a calorie is a calorie."* They want us to believe that fructose—and, by inference, all sugar—is just "empty calories." If it were, then sugar would be the same as—no better, no worse than—any other nutrient. In their view, for a standard sedentary adult consuming 2,000 calories per day, approximately 1,800 calories are "essential" calories, in that they are directed to producing lipids for cell membranes, protein for muscles and enzymes, and carbohydrates for normal energy metabolism, growth, and repair. This leaves about 200 calories per day as "discretionary calories," which can be spent any way we want.[1] And if we exercise, we have the capacity to consume an even higher number of discretionary calories.

If we want to use them all on sugar, then we should have the choice to do so. And we do—and then some.

Figure 16.1 shows the number of calories per day of added sugar eaten by children in different age groups in the United States. The fiftieth percentile consumes between 320 and 350 calories of sugar per day throughout their life span, and the ninetieth percentile consumes above 600 calories. Even the two- to three-year-old age group is consuming an average of 180 calories per day in added sugar. We have far exceeded our discretionary calorie limit; in fact, we've left it in our dust. The food industry continues to add more sugar to processed foods because they can. And they know that when they do, we will buy more (see chapters 5 and 11). Soft drinks account for one third of all the sugar consumed. But other foods that never had sugar before are now busting at the seams from the sugar overload (e.g., yogurt, ketchup).

A Short History of the U.S. Sugar Glut

The U.S. sugar glut is the result of more political distortion and behind-the-scenes manipulation than the 2000 Bush-Gore election. We've always had a

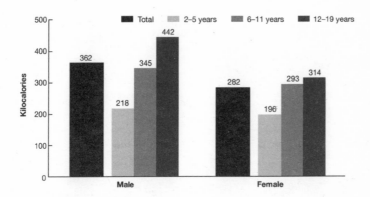

Fig. 16.1a. Sugar in the Morning, Sugar in the Evening, Sugar at Suppertime . . . Daily consumption of added sugars (kilocalories per day) in U.S. children, broken down by age and sex. This comprises all foods, including cereals, desserts, soda, and juice.

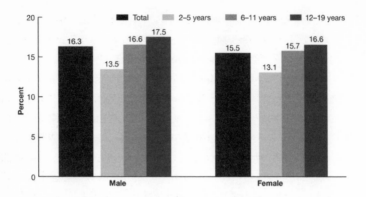

Fig. 16.1b. Daily consumption of added sugars (as a percentage of total calories) in U.S. children, broken down by age and sex. All age groups are consuming more sugar than the upper limit of 10 percent of calories recommended by the American Heart Association.

"sweet tooth," but our consumption of sugar was not a problem until the second half of the twentieth century. North America was consistently a sugar deficit area, requiring more imports than exports to meet growing consumption needs. In chronological order, the events of the past fifty years escalated the problem to bring us to the precipice of our current public health collapse.

1. The Cuban revolution in 1959 and the subsequent assumption of power by Fidel Castro cut off our standard sugar supply. The Bay of Pigs incident in 1961 ended any further dialogue or trade with the Castro regime; we needed a new "sugar fix."

2. High-fructose corn syrup began to hit our shores in the early 1970s. Initially, the U.S. food industry was somewhat wary of this new product. The eventual introduction of HFCS to the Western diet resulted in stability of the U.S. Producer Price Index for sugar because the cost of HFCS, on average, is about half that of sucrose (figure 16.2).

3. President Richard Nixon astutely noted that fluctuating food prices foment political unrest, and he directed his secretary of agriculture, Earl (Rusty) Butz, to "take food off the table" as a politi-

cal issue. Butz's job was to find ways to make food cheap. HFCS fit the bill. This was one of the impetuses for developing the corn subsidy as part of the Farm Bill. Basically, the U.S. government would underwrite the cost of corn, even when it cost more to grow it than to sell it. The low cost of HFCS drove down the price of both, making both substances cheap and readily available.

4. The McGovern Commission (see chapter 10) edict led to a directed policy on the part of the U.S. Department of Agriculture in the late 1970s to reduce our consumption of dietary fat.[2] How do you make low-fat taste good? Add sugar. HFCS was the cheapest alternative around, and homegrown to boot. In the process of switching various processed foods to the low-fat, high-sugar versions, the food industry found that its profits were increasing.

5. The final nail in our coffin came from the second worst hurricane in our history. Everyone remembers Katrina in 2005. Hurricane Allen in 1980 wiped out the entire Caribbean sugar crop in one fell swoop. Sugar futures skyrocketed to $0.55 a pound (a record for that era) and more than $1.00 per pound retail. Coca-Cola, which had been holding out in terms of switching from sucrose to HFCS, now saw a shortage of raw sugar and ushered an HFCS-containing version onto supermarket shelves. The rest of the food industry quickly followed suit.

In the late 1990s, HFCS became the most commonly used sweetener in the United States. Currently, 5 percent of all the corn grown in this country is turned into HFCS.[3] HFCS is no worse for your health than other forms of fructose, though it is always devoid of fiber. However, it's cheap, easy to produce, and readily available—so it now permeates nearly all our food. And we like it, so we buy more. While HFCS is cheaper to produce than sugar, the prices on various foods containing it have remained the same if not gotten higher. (Check out the price of a box of cereal.) A win-win for the food industry.

Influence of corn sweetners on the price of sugar

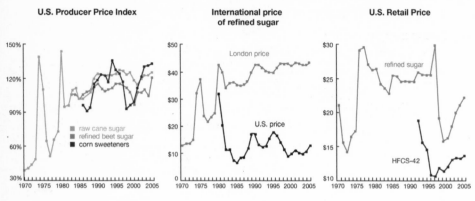

U.S. Department of Agriculture

Fig. 16.2. A Cheap Fix. a) The U.S. producer price index (PPI) for sugar before and after introduction of corn sweeteners in 1975. Upon its introduction, PPI hovers, at 100%, which infers price stability. b) Price of U.S. sugar compared to London price, documenting price stability and allowing for increased usage overseas. c) Price of refined sugar compared to HFCS in the U.S. HFCS was so cheap, it started appearing in every food. And that's where it remains today.

The Food Industry's Justification

The food industry will counter that there are many reasons to add sucrose or HFCS to food and to remove the food's fiber. And some of them are very reasonable, both industrially and economically. But how about biologically? How about in terms of our health?

Sugar Adds Sweetness

Our tongue is able to distinguish five tastes: sweet, salty, sour, bitter, and savory. Sugar covers up the other four. It covers up salty (trail mix, honey roasted peanuts), sour (the acidity in processed tomato sauce provided by less-than-ripe tomatoes, or lemonade), bitter (milk chocolate), and savory (sweet-and-sour pork). Sugar covers up the inequities of foods, making not-so-tasty food seem like it is worth eating. Bottom line, you can make pretty much anything taste good with enough sugar. And the food industry does.

Sugar and Browning

The browning of foods is appealing to your eye and to your taste buds. We slather our ribs in barbecue sauce before we cook or grill them, to get just the right browning effect. All foods brown better with sugar. And the browning of meats provides a smokier, tangier flavor. As discussed in chapter 11, the browning of food is the Maillard reaction.[4] While appealing on the plate and to the palate, it's not so appealing in your arteries.

Sugar Adds Texture

Baked goods wouldn't be nearly as interesting without sugar. Try to make a cake with Splenda. It will taste just as sweet, but it won't puff up. In baked bread, the yeast needs something to work on to give it its airiness. Conversely, wafer crackers wouldn't be crisp if it weren't for sugar. Sugar provides viscosity (thickness) to various foods, such as gummy bears. Sugar also provides the "glass" appearance and crunch of hard candies. Furthermore, sugar lowers foods' freezing point (which is essential for ice cream to have that creamy consistency) and raises their boiling point (which makes caramels chewy).

Sugar Stops Spoilage

Sugar reduces water activity, or the intensity with which water associates with solids. The higher the water activity, the more easily bacteria and mold grow on food. And easily moldy food means quicker spoilage. But sugar (and salt, for that matter) reduces water activity, and makes it less likely that any given food will be able to spoil. This is why the food industry uses sugar as a preservative. When was the last time you tasted a rancid soft drink? Flat maybe, but never rancid. Nothing can grow in that bottle.

The addition of sugar to a food also adds humectancy, which is the ability to hold on to water. This is extremely important for preventing your favorite treats from going stale, particularly your baked goods. One way to gauge the effect of sugar on humectancy is the staling of bread. How long does a loaf of bread purchased at your local bakery take to go stale? About two days. How long does a loaf of commercial bread purchased at the supermarket take to go stale? About two to three weeks. This works for the consumer because it retards spoilage and reduces waste. The food industry and the supermarket associations are happy because it reduces depreciation, thereby increasing profits. I checked my local supermarket: of the thirty-two commercially available breads there, thirty-one were made with HFCS, added for both browning and humectancy. And what were they lacking? Fiber.

Fast Food and Fiber

Currently, the median U.S. fiber consumption is 12 grams per day. This is on purpose. The food industry removes fiber from food because fiber limits shelf life. Bread devoid of fiber is going to last far longer in your pantry than if you buy it fresh at the farmers' market. And the food industry capitalizes on this. Reduced depreciation means reduced costs, which means increased sales. What's the definition of *fast food*? It's fiberless food. Because you can't freeze fiber and expect to maintain the same texture. Fiberless food can be frozen, shipped globally, and cooked quickly. But getting rid of fiber has obviated satiety, and exacerbated the negative impact of the carbohydrates, contributing to hyperinsulinemia, obesity, and metabolic syndrome.

When You Can't Justify, Deflect

So there you are. Lots of reasons to add sugar and remove fiber. Good for the visual presentation. Good for the palate. Good for the pocketbook. Good for the industry. But bad for your health. Let's take a generic cookie as an example: 30 percent flour, 30 percent fat, 30 percent sugar, and about 6 percent protein. This is the ultimate concoction of fat and carbohydrate possible in one food item. And sweetness has more salience (appeal) when you add fat. (Which would you rather eat: Pixie Stix or a Cinnabon?) One cookie is a treat. But bet you can't eat just one, because sugar is addictive, and sugar plus fat is even more so. Our caloric overload, generated specifically by added sugars, proves it.

The food industry says they do not understand what all the fuss is about. Sugar has been around for millennia. Sugar is a source of energy. Sugar is a "natural" part of our diet. True, but irrelevant in terms of our health. Here are some samples of the claims the food industry or their ambassadors have used to persuade the public that the addition of added sugar to food or drinks is as American as apple pie (with extra HFCS).

Food Industry Argument #1: Fructose Doesn't Raise Blood Glucose

The industry argues that fructose doesn't raise blood glucose, and they're right. Fructose has a very low glycemic index (see chapters 11 and 17), which is a measure of a food's generation of an insulin response and is used as a method for quantifying a food's potential for weight gain. But remember, there's no fructose alone in nature. It is always found with glucose (either as sucrose or HFCS), and the glucose contribution generates quite a hefty insulin response.[5] So when the glucose is metabolized, it drives up insulin, while the fructose causes liver fat and liver insulin resistance. Carbohydrates and fat together. A great way to get metabolic syndrome.

Food Industry Argument #2: Switch 'Em Up: Fructose for Glucose

The food industry would like to develop crystalline fructose (alone) as an FDA-approved sweetener. They base this idea on several "controlled" studies that demonstrate that when you substitute fructose for glucose (calorie for calorie) there is no rise in HbA_{1c} (what doctors test the blood for in order to assess blood sugar control in diabetic patients), a fact that suggests that fructose would be desirable for diabetics.[6] Perhaps one reason for this is that crystalline fructose is incompletely absorbed by the small intestine, and thus its effects on glucose and HbA_{1c} may be minimal. However, if your body doesn't absorb the crystalline fructose, the GI symptoms caused by the residual fructose wreak havoc on the intestine, generating pain, bloating, and diarrhea.[7] Remember how Olestra was going to revolutionize America? As a fat substitute, it purported to add no fat, calories, or cholesterol to products. True, but it quickly lost its market share due to side effects. As described by the health warning label, "This product contains

Olestra. Olestra may cause abdominal cramping and loose stools. Olestra inhibits the absorption of some vitamins and other nutrients." The additive quickly became synonymous with "anal leakage" and has since disappeared. Crystalline fructose may follow the same path.

Furthermore, just because fructose doesn't raise HbA_{1c} levels in the bloodstream of diabetics, that doesn't mean it's not doing damage; Japanese researchers have shown that fructose binds to proteins in people.[8] It also doesn't mean that fructose is not doing damage to proteins *inside* cells. Studies of animals receiving ad lib sucrose versus starch show marked inflammation of liver cells leading to cirrhosis.[9] Likewise, studies of humans have demonstrated that sucrose consumption correlates with the degree of liver inflammation.

The food industry points to controlled studies in which fructose is substituted for glucose, with no increase in weight. (After all, if the calories eaten are the same, then one would expect this.)[10] They also like to quote a famous 1999 study showing that the liver turns fructose to fat at a very low rate (less than 5 percent).[11] If you believe this, you should be able to drink as much soda as you want! Not so fast. It holds true only if you're thin, fasting (and therefore glycogen depleted), and given fructose alone (which is poorly absorbed). Rather, if you're obese, insulin-resistant, fed, and getting both fructose and glucose together (a sizeable percentage of the population), then fructose gets converted to fat at a much higher rate, approximating 25 percent. In other words, the toxicity of fructose depends on the context. If you're an elite athlete and glycogen-depleted, you can eat or drink pretty much anything you want. But if you're not, then our current excessive sugar supply doesn't work for you.

Food Industry Argument #3: The Food Label Is Right There!

The food industry argues that the information on sugar and fiber in our food is right there on the Nutrition Facts label, in plain sight, for all to see. Based on that information, people can make their own conscious decisions. Not quite. Under the carbohydrate heading, the Nutrition Facts label lists "total sugars." This signifies a combination of all versions of monosaccharides, which include glucose, fructose, and galactose (milk sugar); and all disaccharides, which include maltose (glucose-glucose, found in beer), lactose (glucose-galactose, found in dairy), and sucrose (glucose-fructose, found everywhere!). For instance, one cup of low-fat milk has 12 grams of sugar, which comes from lactose. The galactose is not a problem, as it is metabolized to glucose and does not pose a significant health threat, unless you have the disease galactosemia, in which case you'd have died of an overwhelming infection before you were two months old.

Furthermore, the fructose that is found naturally in many foods is also not a problem. This amount is usually small, and invariably there is some associated fiber, which limits its negative effects. "All-natural" juice may not contain added sugar, but because the fiber has ben removed from it (see chapter 12), it's just a sugar-sweetened beverage. Again, ounce for ounce, juice has more fructose and more calories than soft drinks. What about canned fruit? The fruit itself is fine, but they can't add water to the can, because the sugar in the fruit would leach out. They instead add sugar syrup in high concentration, to keep the fruit sweet and soft and to prevent spoilage. It's the "added sugar" that we need to know about, which is always either sucrose or HFCS, put in the food specifically by the food industry for palatability and shelf life. Likewise, we need to know how much fiber is included and how much has been removed.

But you're not allowed to know this. The Nutrition Labeling and Education Act (NLEA) of 1990 allows for the declaration of "total sugars" as a whole.[12] There is no differentiation between them or provision for "added sugars." The FDA stated that there was no scientific evidence to argue that the body makes any distinction between natural or added sugar. The inclusion of "added sugars" in the label underrepresents the sugar content of foods high in endogenous or natural sugars. However, the fiber is the mitigating factor, not the sugar. Lastly, the FDA believes there would be no way to enforce such a rule and that the food industry would have no impetus to conform to it. But the real reason we're not allowed to know is pressure from food industry lobbyists. Their argument to the FDA in 1989 was, "If we listed the added sugars on the label, then all our competitors could duplicate our recipes. This is proprietary information, and we won't release it." And the FDA bought that argument. Do you? You may not believe the premise, but you buy the products.

You'll also notice that there are Recommended Daily Values for every one of the other nutrients on the food label. But there is no Recommended Daily Value or Dietary Reference Intake (DRI) for sugar, either natural or added. I recently had the occasion to sit on a panel with Sam Kass, Michelle Obama's personal chef and her pointman to the White House Childhood Obesity Task Force. I asked him straight out, "Why is there no DRI for sugar?" His response might surprise you: "Why would you need a DRI for something that is not a nutrient?" Wow! Sugar is not a nutrient? That might be news to the USDA. I actually kind of agree with Mr. Kass. Sugar is certainly not an essential nutrient, in the sense that there is not one single biochemical reaction that requires it. Sugar is extraneous, and our bodies certainly don't need it. As elaborated in chapter 11, sugar is more toxin than it ever was a nutrient.

Food Industry Argument #4: It's All About Supply and Demand

There are two philosophies of marketing, and the food industry has mastered both.

1. *We give the public what it wants.* The food industry is just responding to a need by filling a "niche" in the American economy. This is how the industry would like to be portrayed—as "reactive." Portion sizes in this country are significantly larger than they were twenty years ago. You buy a larger portion because you feel you're getting a better deal. You buy more, you eat more. Everybody wins. Well, not everybody. The food industry wins by selling more, the middleman wins by levying the markup, the government wins by levying the sales tax. You lose.

2. *If you build it, they will come.* This is the real story: developing a market out of nowhere—or being "proactive." As I like to tell my children, "Advertising is necessary only for products that we don't want and don't need." The food industry (manufacturers, retailers, and food service) is outranked only by the automobile industry in terms of monetary expenditure for marketing. Like it or not, we are influenced in our choices by what the media tell us to want. Especially our children. You may "know" that you should eat more fruits and vegetables, but how many commercials do you

or your kids watch that say so? Less than 5 percent of all food advertising dollars is spent by the fruit, vegetable, and grain sectors. The government and USDA can't compete with the almost unlimited funds of the food industry. In 1997 the USDA spent $300 million to promote healthy eating, in comparison to the $11 billion spent advertising junk food, of which $4.2 billion was directed at children[13] (see chapter 20).

Grease Their Palms to Grease the Wheels

That fast food and beverage companies sponsor teams, sporting events, charity walks, and other physical activity–related venues to take the heat off the sugar they peddle is as American as apple pie. It's another thing entirely for them to finance the uniforms and the scoreboards for schools around the country. In exchange for financial compensation, schools sign exclusive marketing contracts with beverage companies to permit on-campus advertising through product donations, scoreboards and signs, clothing, and school supplies. The more beverages sold, the more money for the school and more profits for the company. In a 2000 survey, 72 percent of California high schools allowed advertising for fast food and beverages on campus, while only 13 percent prohibited it. And if you think it's bad in the United States, try Latin America. Consumption of soft drinks doubled in Mexico in seven years. Despite the fact that 75 percent of Mexican adults are currently overweight, Coca-Cola sponsors more physical activity programs than all other companies put together.[14]

If You Can't Beat 'Em, Join 'Em

Despite the rhetoric, the food industry knows it has a problem. Enter the new market of "functional foods." As Pepsico chairwoman Indra Nooyi so eloquently stated in *The New Yorker* (May 16, 2011), "It's not a question of selling less. It's a question of selling the right stuff." In response to the obesity pandemic, Pepsi now has three lines: "Fun for you" (e.g., chips and soda), "Better for you" (e.g., juice and beef jerky), and "Good for you" (e.g., whole grains, fruits, vegetables, low-fat dairy, nuts).

Americans know that they're gaining weight and that they should be eating healthier. So the food industry helps us assuage our guilt with processed products labeled "natural" and "whole wheat," or containing "extra nutrients." You buy them, probably paying extra, and feel better about eating them. None of these taglines has any meaningful definition, and there is little to no regulation about when they can be used. We are currently in "throwback" mode: many soft drink manufacturers, such as Pepsi, are substituting sucrose for HFCS based on the myth that sucrose is more "natural" and therefore better for you. Sobe Drinks, with 100 percent of your daily vitamin C requirements, are essentially sugar water, with vitamin C added to make you think you're getting more for your money. Just because you don't feel any guilt doesn't mean your body won't feel the effects. Promise—if all the HFCS-containing candy bars in the world somehow mysteriously were replaced by their sucrose-containing equivalents, they would still be junk food, and your body wouldn't know the difference—although they might cost more and you might balk at the increased price.

Investors are watching Pepsi carefully. As it promotes its "Good for You" line, it has reduced the marketing of its "Fun for You" line, to the tune of $349 million. In the process, Pepsi-Cola has fallen to third place in soft drink sales, behind Coke and Diet Coke. It remains to be seen if what is essentially a "junk food company" can recreate itself. If not, don't expect any risk taking from the others.

Who's in Charge?

If there's any lesson to be gleaned from this book, it's that food is health. But while you are ostensibly in charge of your health, you are clearly not in charge of your food. In fact, those who are in charge of your food are doing their level best to make a buck off you. Food companies in the year 2010 generated nearly $1 trillion in sales. And if your health goes down the tubes, that's your problem. But it's not just *your* problem. It's everyone's problem. The cigarette industry was chastised for an irrational business model: poisoning your best customers is not considered a growth strategy. But if you can hook more people on the front end, you can guarantee your supply of users, so you can afford to lose a few. The food industry has a leg up on this model: corner the food market, and people will have no place else to go. Is it any wonder that the food industry, in the midst of two negative trends—the economic downturn and the obesity pandemic—is making money hand over fist?

PART V

The Personal Solution

Chapter 17

Altering Your Food Environment

———————•———————

John was born at normal weight, but with a voracious appetite, and became massively obese by age one. By fifteen, he was up to 340 pounds. His parents sent him to the Academy of the Sierras ("fat school") for a year, where his food was restricted and his weight dropped by 100 pounds. Within three months of returning home, he gained 140 pounds. He then came to see me. Genetic testing showed that he had two mutations in the gene coding for a protein that mediates the satiety signal in the hypothalamus. In other words, his hunger, appetite, and obesity were due to a genetic defect. Nonetheless, when his environment was controlled, even he could lose weight.

As this clinical vignette shows us, controlling behavior doesn't work, because behavior is really just the output of our biochemistry. Controlling behavior is unsustainable. If your brain can't receive the leptin signal (see chapters 4–6), it thinks it's being starved and it initiates behaviors to regain the weight. But even John, a patient with a genetic defect, can lose weight when his environment is controlled and his access to food is regulated (although there are rare exceptions, as with the brain tumor children). The problem is how to control our environment adequately, when there is such free access to high-sugar, low-fiber food, to help us with our weight. Parents can do so—they must make their homes safe for their children (see chapter 18). Our culture needs to adopt the precept that making a home safe for a toddler includes both child safety locks and a wholesome food environment. But once a child enters puberty—a state of insulin resistance, independence, allowance, and peer pressure—the game is over. That's why virtually all anti-obesity interventions work better in younger children.

Our environment is toxic (see chapters 10–15) because it is insulinogenic and, in turn, obesogenic.[1] For the vast majority of obese people, in order to reverse the process, the goal is to *get the insulin down*. That starts with what you eat, and it means altering your point of contact—your relationship with your supermarket, grocery store, and restaurants.

"Trash Talk" on the Dietary Playground

The public is preoccupied and yet completely flummoxed by the low-fat-versus-low-carb diet controversy. They couldn't be further apart both on the evolutionary scene and in the supermarket, where the meat and produce aisles are located on opposite sides of the store. The proponents of each of these diets aggressively dispute the others. Today, there are more authors in this arena than any other aspect of health. Scientists "trash-talk" their opponents, as if bringing the other side down will elevate one's cause. Medical societies have taken sides. Their venom has created a noxious atmosphere. The fallout from this "food fight" has confused the issue and given the entire discipline of nutrition a bad name.

The "Dish" on Diets

Most people will put themselves "on a diet" in an attempt to lose weight, ostensibly by controlling their food environment. But what does this mean? Why do these diets work for some but not for others? What's the most rational diet for you? Do any of them perform as advertised? There are more fad diets than there are cold remedies. Furthermore, when a diet doesn't work, the assumption is that you weren't compliant with it. But compliance is a measure of change in behavior. Sustainable behavior change means changing the environment.

To pry behavior and environment apart, first let's start with the basic precepts of what makes a good diet. As an example, let's examine a "failed" diet and determine why it failed.

The Low-Fat Diet—a Dismal Failure

As discussed in chapter 10, the low-fat diet is what got us into this mess. It started out as a prescription to prevent heart disease, not obesity. The link between dietary fat and heart disease is based on findings regarding a genetic disease called familial hypercholesterolemia (FH), which affects 1 percent of the population.[2] In the 1980s the low-fat diet became the diet recommended by every health organization in America (AHA, both ADAs [American Diabetes *and* Dietetic associations], the National Heart, Lung, and Blood Institute, and so on) to control obesity as well as prevent heart disease. Their mantra was eating less fat would reduce the total number of calories and contribute to weight loss because *a calorie is a calorie*. Except it's not.

So what happened to the other 99 percent of the population? Does the low-fat diet work for them? As the Occupy Wall Street movement says, the other 99 percent got screwed. Not only does it not work in the way it is routinely employed, but it is likely detrimental for three different reasons. First, a low-fat diet tastes like cardboard; the flavor is in the fat. So you up the carbs to compensate, increasing your insulin, and your weight (see chapter 9). Second, as discussed in chapter 10, there are two LDLs. Large buoyant (type A) LDL, which accounts for about 80 percent of the circulating LDL, is increased by saturated fat. But large buoyant LDL has a neutral impact and by itself poses little risk for heart disease. Conversely, small dense (type B) LDL, which accounts for the other 20 percent, is driven by dietary carbohydrates.[3] It is type B that contributes to heart disease.[4] Third, if dietary fats were merely sources of energy, then we wouldn't have a class of essential fatty acids that we literally cannot live without. We need to eat certain dietary fats for our nervous system and immune systems, cell membranes, and to make certain hormones. So you have a choice: you can eat good fats in your diet or you can make bad ones in your liver. Wouldn't you rather opt for the good ones?

The reason the low-fat diet is a dismal failure is explained by the science in chapters 10–12. It's not the fat, it's not the carbohydrate—it's the fat *and* the carbohydrate together that cause metabolic problems. Sugar provides just that, and the low-fat diet is rife with it. The lack of fiber in the processed low-fat diet means that the rate of flux of both fat and carbohydrates to the liver is heightened, putting your poor liver under even more stress. The epitome of failure.

As you will see, all successful diets share three precepts: low sugar, high fiber (which means high micronutrients), and fat and carbohydrate consumed together in the presence of an offsetting amount of fiber. Anything after that is window dressing.

The Atkins Diet—Depends on How It's Done

The adherents to the low-carb diet are numerous because, for the most part, it does work for weight loss and improved metabolic health.[5] The most famous of the low-carb options is the Atkins diet, which says, "Bring on the bratwurst, banish the bun." Indeed, the Atkins diet is one, albeit somewhat radical, method for treating the co-morbidities of metabolic syndrome. The question is, does the Atkins diet work because it is low-carb, or because it is low-sugar? We still don't know.

Four issues complicate the use of the Atkins diet as a full-time regime. First, a fat is not a fat (see chapter 10). The quality of the fat counts, and scarfing down bad ones can also be detrimental. Second, the Atkins diet says you should eat your vegetables, especially the green ones, but casual Atkins dabblers don't—that's why they *like* the diet. But the vegetables confer both fiber and micronutrients (see chapter 12). One animal model suggests that despite weight loss, the Atkins diet can increase other risk factors for atherosclerosis.[6] Furthermore, the diet can result in inadequacies in the micronutrients thiamine, folic acid, vitamin C, iron, and magnesium, all of which could have been supplied with the fiber.[7] The Atkins diet cuts out milk because lactose is a carbohydrate—there goes the vitamin D for your bone health. And the higher protein forces urinary calcium loss, putting your bones at greater risk. Third, many people gauge the success of the Atkins diet by their degree of weight loss. However, that's because most of the early weight loss is due to loss of liver and muscle glycogen, which is sur-rounded by water molecules. But this is a double-edged sword, because even a minor transgression will form new glycogen, bringing water with it. Fourth, adherence to the Atkins diet is very uneven.[8] And good luck trying to keep a kid on the Atkins diet during the school year. The question is, do you really need to be this extreme? Isn't there a better way?

The Vegetarian/Vegan Diet—Depends on How It's Done

What about the opposite? As you saw from the case of Sujatha in chapter 12's clinical vignette, eating vegan or vegetarian is no protection against obesity or metabolic syndrome. Processed foods devoid of animal products can be just as bad for you as those containing them. Because any diet can be processed, with the removal of fiber and the addition of fat, carbohydrates, and sugar, just as easily as the Western diet. So it's all in the execution. If you eat a vegetarian or vegan diet the way our gatherer ancestors did—eating the food as it comes out of the ground—you're good to go, although you might need to supplement the diet with calcium and vitamin D. But if you eat the "processed" vegetarian diet out of the middle shelves of the su-permarket, with fat and sugar additives for palatability and the removal of fiber for shelf life,[9] then you and Sujatha's mother can wallow in your incre-dulity together.

The Traditional Japanese Diet

The *traditional* Japanese diet is polished white rice (lots of carbohydrate), a little fish, some fermented soybeans, and lots of vegetables. And it works in preventing both obesity and chronic metabolic disease. (I should men-tion that the *modern* Japanese diet, replete with HFCS, is just as bad as the U.S. diet. Japanese are getting metabolic syndrome in record numbers and are doing bariatric surgery at Tokyo Children's Hospital.) Even though it is high in carbs, the traditional Japanese diet works for four reasons: First, there is virtually no sugar to promote insulin resistance. Second, the insu-lin rise caused by the glucose in the rice is partially attenuated by the fiber in their vegetables. Third, the fish is high in omega-3s. Four, it's high in micronutrients and antioxidants. A winning combination. Using fiber as the antidote to carbohydrate (see chapter 12) is the salvation of many a successful diet.

The Mediterranean Diet

Pioppi, a small town in Italy, is the home of the Mediterranean diet. In Ancel Keys' Seven Countries study (Italy was one the countries), this diet was associated with lower death rates from heart disease. The diet was popularized in America due to its population's low incidence of disease and long lifespan. Unfortunately, Pioppi and many surrounding areas that originally consumed a peasant fare can no longer afford to do so. Processed food is more readily available and cheaper. These areas, once renowned for their health, have soaring rates of obesity in part due to a current lack of whole grains, fresh fruits, and vegetables from their diets. These items are just too expensive, and they don't taste as good.

Here's what's in the *real* Mediterranean diet: high olive oil consumption (monounsaturated fat); legumes (beans, lentils, peas); fruits, vegetables, and unrefined grains (fiber); dairy products (saturated fat); eggs (high-quality protein); fish (omega-3s); and wine in moderation (resveratrol, flavonoids, and likely other factors).[10] Americans misunderstand the Mediterranean diet, because they think it is all about pasta, which is Italian but *not* Mediterranean. Because what the Italians used to eat in Italy is not what the Italians ate in the United States. The pasta and pizza movement actually started in the United States within the poor Italian immigrant population, based on the cost of carbohydrates versus meat. That diet then migrated over to Italy. And now the Italians have our problem.

The Ornish Diet

This diet, popularized by Dean Ornish at the University of California, San Francisco in his 1993 book, *Eat More, Weigh Less*, is the one diet that has been proven not only to promote weight loss but to *reverse heart disease* and improve cellular health, hypothetically increasing your lifespan.[11] The Ornish diet espouses that participants should not get more than 10 percent of their calories from fat. (A low-fat diet provides about 30 percent of calories as fat.)

Here's what's allowed on the Ornish diet: beans and legumes, fruits, whole grains, and vegetables (in other words, all fiber all the time). Ornish allows nonfat dairy products in moderation. And here are the no-nos: meat of all kinds, poultry, oils and oil-containing products (e.g., salad dressings), nuts and seeds, sugar, and alcohol. In other words, the no-fun diet. Ornish decries anything with a saturated fat or an omega-6, which is highly defensible. But he is conflicted on the consumption of fish. While he acknowledges that fish is rich in omega-3s, which can reduce sudden cardiac death by 50–80 percent, he'd rather take fish oil capsules. He argues that eating salmon, mackerel, halibut, and other deepwater fishes provides a lot of extra fat and cholesterol, along with mercury and other toxic waste products that have found their way into the ocean. Ornish also has a love-hate relationship with olive oil, which provides oleic acid, a stimulator of an important liver health pathway. But he chides that olive oil is 14 percent saturated fat and 100 percent total fat. So, the more olive oil consumed, the higher your cholesterol goes.

As far as I am concerned, that's throwing the baby out with the bathwater. The low-fat diet, promoted by the government and doctors in the 1980s and 1990s, failed because it didn't tell you what else to eat and what to restrict. As Ornish clearly shows, fat by itself is not the culprit; it's what you substitute for it that causes the problem. But the biggest problem is that when adherents are left to the whim of the grocery store, the Ornish diet gradually morphs into the general low-fat diet, with all its problems.[12]

The Paleolithic Diet—an Evolutionary Compromise

The Paleolithic diet, which is low-carb and high-fat, includes foods that were available to our ancestors prior to agriculture: meat, fish, nuts, natural fruits, and vegetables. It excludes milk, grains, and processed foods of any sort. This diet has been popularized by scientists, including Loren Cordain and S. Boyd Eaton.[13] Staffan Lindeberg studied the inhabitants of Kitava, an island just off Papua New Guinea, who still live naturally on this diet today.[14] They do not suffer from heart disease, diabetes, obesity, hypertension, or stroke. My UCSF colleague Dr. Lynda Frassetto has shown that even ten days of a Paleolithic diet can improve blood pressure, insulin sensitivity, glucose tolerance, and lipid profiles whether or not you lose weight.[15] One issue with the Paleolithic diet is the lack of vitamin D and calcium (not an issue for our Paleolithic ancestors, who spent all their time outdoors), which could potentially be made up with supplements. Others knock its reliance on animal meat as a protein source, but the quality of the fats is still much better than with the Western diet. This diet also excludes all grains, including those with fiber, which may not be necessary to limit. But perhaps the biggest problem is its expense. To do this diet right costs way more than a trip to Whole Foods, which means that the poor aren't invited to the Caveman Party.

The Low–Glycemic Index Diet—Theory versus Practice

Another alternative for reducing insulin that has procured press and adherents is called the low–glycemic index (GI) diet. "Glycemic index" refers to a theory of eating with the purpose of keeping down blood sugar (and therefore insulin), but it is not the panacea that the zealots hype. GI is a simple concept: how high does your serum glucose rise in response to 50 grams of carbohydrate in any given food, as compared with the glucose response in 50 grams of straight starch (white bread). However, as we saw in chapter 8, it's not the glucose response that matters; it's the insulin response that follows. The yo-yo glucose-insulin effect of a high-GI diet is thought to drive excess energy intake and promote obesity.[16]

As useful a concept as GI is, the concept of glycemic load (GL) is even more relevant; it takes into account the beneficial effect of fiber.[17] The GL of a food is calculated as its GI x the amount of that food containing 50 grams of carbohydrate. More fiber means a larger portion, because there's less digestible carbohydrate. You can turn a high-GI food into a low-GL food by eating it with the original fiber. A good example is carrots, which are high-GI (lots of carbohydrates) but low-GL (even more fiber).

There are two problems with GI and GL. The low-GI diet is most effective in patients who have obesity due to excessive insulin release by the pancreas.[18] That makes sense based on how the low-GI diet prevents the blood glucose from rising in response to a meal. The second problem with the concepts of GI and GL is fructose itself. Fructose isn't glucose; when eaten, it doesn't raise the glucose and it doesn't raise the insulin directly. Indeed, fructose was originally touted as an excellent sugar alternative for patients with diabetes, precisely because it has a low GI of 20. But fructose is the most egregious cause of liver insulin resistance and metabolic syndrome, because of its unique liver metabolism (see chapter 11). This hasn't stopped the food industry from trying to capitalize on the low-GI craze by adding fructose to foods. The low-GL diet takes into account insulin suppression and fiber. Add to that a low-fructose diet, and you have the main tenets of the South Beach diet. Keeping insulin low, eating lots of fiber, and avoiding added sugar. Now you've got something.

Tweaking Your Diet Based on Genetics or Biochemistry

Should our genetics determine our diet? Some diets may work better in one person or another based on genetics. Certainly, for the 1 percent with familial hypercholesterolemia (see chapter 10), it's either the low-fat diet (with statins) or Heart Attack City. Latinos are famous for developing diabetes and nonalcoholic fatty liver disease, due to a gene alteration expressed in the liver. If you're one of the 19 percent of Latinos with this gene defect, then any fructose you consume goes straight to liver fat—do not pass Go, do not collect $200. And in one study, the success of different diets was dependent on three separate genes that control fat metabolism.[19]

By far and away, your insulin profile is the most important factor in determining what diet approach will work best for you. Here are four different studies that argue for knowing your insulin:

1. The low-GI diet worked best in those subjects whose pancreases released the most insulin.[20]
2. The low-carb diet worked best in the subjects with the most insulin resistance.[21]
3. Yet, if the insulin resistance is caused by a genetic variation, then

going low-carb can't fix the problem, in which case a high-carb,
low-fat diet is more effective in improving weight loss.[22]

4.   And of course, our octreotide studies (see chapter 4) argue that
insulin suppression is an effective method to promote weight loss.

Commonsense Dieting Means *No* Dieting

Let's look at all these diets. Some rely on fat for energy, others rely on carbohydrates for energy, and some use both. Yet they all work to control
weight and improve metabolic health, and have been shown to reduce heart
disease. What do they all share? Two things. They are all low in sugar, and
they are all high in fiber (and therefore high in micronutrients). We've arrived. That's the point—that's what matters. You now hold the keys to the
kingdom. Naturally occurring fructose comes from sugarcane, fruits, some
vegetables, and honey. The first three have way more fiber than fructose,
and the last is protected by bees. Nature made sugar hard to get. Man made
it easy to get. And that's the nugget of truth that the food industry and the
U.S. government won't admit; because if they did, they'd have to scale back,
and they either can't or don't want to (see chapter 21). That's why the rates
of obesity and chronic metabolic disease have skyrocketed wherever the
industrial global diet has been introduced.

The number of people who can stick to any diet is exceedingly small.
Recidivism is the watchword of dieting. First there's temptation. Then there's
convenience. Then there's lack of access. Then there's boredom. And the
"cherry on the frappe" is the negative-weight plateau for most dieters,
which weakens your willpower even further.

Diet Sweeteners: Panacea or Propaganda?

This is one of the thorniest issues in nutrition today. On this subject, I am
agnostic—because the data on which to make a recommendation on which
diet sweetener is best, or on whether diet sweeteners are a smart alternative
at all, remain elusive.

Diet sweeteners, on the surface, would make perfect sense as an alternative to either sucrose or HFCS. They substitute sweetness for calories and remove the offending fructose. The United States has been slowly but surely turning to diet drinks because of the obesity epidemic; as of 2010, 42 percent of Coca-Cola sales in the United States were of the diet variety. Not so fast. If 33 percent of all sugar consumption is in drinks, and 42 percent of drinks are now diet, someone should be losing weight. Yet there is not one study that shows that substituting diet drinks for sugared ones actually causes weight loss in obese subjects. There are several studies, promoted by the sugar industry, that demonstrate that consumption of diet drinks correlates with the prevalence of metabolic syndrome.[23] But remember, correlation is not causation. Do diet sweeteners cause metabolic syndrome, or do people with metabolic syndrome consume more diet drinks to assuage their guilt from eating Twinkies? So why don't we know if the substitution of diet sweeteners for sugar actually reduces caloric intake, body fat, and metabolic disease?[24] There are five specific issues that underlie our ignorance.[25]

1. There is a difference between pharmacokinetics and pharmacodynamics. In short, pharmacokinetics is what your body does to a drug; pharmacodynamics is what a drug does to your body. They are not the same—far from it. We have all the information on pharmacokinetics for all the diet sweeteners to determine safety, because the FDA demands it before any sweetener is approved for the U.S. market. But we have none of the pharmacodynamics. We don't know what any of these diet sweeteners do to your long-term food intake, weight, body fat, or metabolic status. And the reason we don't have the pharmacodynamics is that the FDA doesn't demand such studies. They examine only two criteria for a drug (or sweetener) to be approved: safety and efficacy. So the food industry doesn't do the studies because such studies are expensive and may have detrimental effects on sales. And the NIH won't do them, saying it's the food industry's job. So the studies don't get done. What about the nonabsorbed sweeteners? Sugar alcohols such as xylitol and sorbitol aren't absorbed across the intestine, so they're safe, right? Yes, except that in high amounts they cause significant gastrointestinal distress, bloating, and diarrhea.

2.   Here's a hypothetical concern. You drink a soda. The tongue tastes either sugar or diet sweetener—it doesn't know which—and sends the "sweet" signal to the hypothalamus, which says, "Hey, a sugar load is coming, get ready to metabolize it." The hypothalamus then sends a signal along the vagus nerve to the pancreas, saying, "A sugar load is coming, get ready to release extra insulin." If the "sweet" signal is from a diet sweetener, the sugar never comes. What happens next? Does the hypothalamus say, "Oh, well . . . I'll just chill until the next meal," or does it say, "WTF? I'm all primed for the extra sugar. I'll go find some." We don't know if the brain compensates for the lack of sugar.

3.   The possibility exists that diet sweeteners might change the composition of intestinal bacteria. This may generate inflammation (see chapter 12), and increase deposition of visceral fat.

4.   We don't know the role that diet sweeteners may play in sugar addiction (see chapter 5). Down-regulation of dopamine receptors by sucrose means you have to supply more sugar next time to get the same effect, creating a positive feedback system and driving further intake. The same has been seen with diet sweeteners. So, conceivably, diet sweeteners foment the same biochemical dependence, which drives further sugar-seeking behavior. So even if you don't get sugar at this meal, you'll make sure you get it at the next one.

5.   The issue of diet sweetener safety is extremely complex. The FDA party line says, if it's approved, it's safe. But is it? Concerns continue to abound about aspartame, despite its availability on the market for the past thirty years. Then there's the other side. The sugar industry has loads of reasons for blurring the landscape. Any diet sweetener that threatens their dominance generates a no-holds-barred takedown. They've attacked every diet sweetener that has appeared on the market since saccharine.

How to Navigate a Food Label

Controlling your personal food environment is all about the point of decision. How do you navigate your supermarket? It's a minefield.

First Rule

If you go to the market hungry, all is lost.

Second Rule

Shop on the periphery of the supermarket. If you go into the shelves, you've gone off the ranch.

Third Rule

Real food doesn't have or need a Nutrition Facts label. The more labels you read, the more garbage you're buying.

Fourth Rule

Real food spoils—which is a good thing. If bacteria can digest it, that means you can, too (since your mitochondria are just repurposed bacteria). There are three major downsides to eating real food. The first is that it takes time to cook. But by eating real food, you automatically increase your levels of fiber and micronutrients and reduce your fructose and trans fats. The second is that it spoils, so you can't keep it in your pantry indefinitely. The third is that real food is more expensive. That's the biggest problem.

Fifth Rule

Find the hidden sugar. And they hide it well. The Nutrition Facts label requires the listing of ingredients by mass. By using different forms of sugar in any given product, the food industry can add many different sugars to one product. The grams don't change, but the order on the label does. The food industry has at least forty other names for sugar, in an effort to hide it on the label, but a discerning eye can always spot them (table 17.1). Caveat emptor (buyer beware)!

Table 17.1. Various Names for Sugar Added to Processed Foods

Agave nectar*	Barbados sugar*	Barley malt	Beet sugar*
Blackstrap molasses*	Brown sugar*	Buttered syrup*	Cane juice crystals*
Cane sugar*	Caramel*	Carob syrup*	Castor sugar*
Confectioner's sugar*	Corn syrup	Corn syrup solids	Crystalline fructose*
Date sugar*	Demerara sugar*	Dextran	Dextrose
Diastatic malt	Diatase	Ethyl maltol	Evaporated cane juice*
Florida crystals*	Fructose*	Fruit juice*	Fruit juice concentrate*
Galactose	Glucose	Glucose solids	Golden sugar*
Golden syrup*	Grape sugar*	High-fructose corn syrup*	Honey*
Icing sugar*	Invert sugar*	Lactose	Malt syrup
Maltodextrin	Maltose	Maple syrup*	Molasses*
Muscovado sugar*	Organic raw sugar*	Panocha*	Raw sugar*
Refiner's syrup*	Rice syrup	Sorghum syrup*	Sucrose*
Sugar*	Treacle*	Turbinado sugar*	Yellow sugar*

*Contains fructose.

Plus, the food industry is introducing sugar to infants at an ever-earlier age. Abbott Labs makes Isomil, a lactose-free baby formula; the lactose is substituted with 10.3 percent sucrose. (A Coke is 10.5 percent sucrose.) Mead Johnson discontinued production of their chocolate-flavored "toddler formula" Enfagrow in 2010 because of the backlash from consumers regarding the amount of sugar required to balance the choco-late (which is inherently bitter); however, the vanilla version is still on the market. According to the Center for Science in the Public Interest, Gerber and Heinz add sugars and/or starchy fillers to more than half of their second- and third-stage fruits and several second-stage vegetables. Is it any wonder we have an epidemic of obese six-month olds?

So how to curb your sugar consumption? Start with eliminating all sugared beverages. We were designed to *eat* our calories, not drink them. Just think of a soda as a "fructose delivery vehicle," similar to cigarettes. And juice is worse than soda. Juice has 5.8 teaspoons of sugar per cup; soda has 5.4. Eat your fruit, don't drink it. Second, take all your recipes and wherever sugar is called for, reduce the amount by one third. I promise, your home-baked goods will be better tasting and better for you. You can actually taste the chocolate, the oatmeal, the nuts. Lastly, make dessert special. When I grew up, dessert was once a week. Now it's once a meal and also at snack time. My children know that a weekday dessert means a piece of fruit, and weekends are reserved for something more elaborate. I guarantee you, they won't feel deprived.

If a food has a Nutrition Facts label, by definition it's processed. Everyone immediately focuses on the total calories and grams of saturated fat. These are the least important properties of any food. Here's the real scoop on what to look for on a Nutrition Facts label: If it's a liquid, it should have 5 calories or less. (Unflavored milk is the only exception. Remember, milk sugar is lactose, which turns into glucose in the liver—no fructose here.) If it's a solid, it should have 3 grams of fiber or more (See chapter 12). If the words *partially hydrogenated* (aka trans fat) appear anywhere, it's been designed not to go rancid. So it may very well outlast you. If any form of sugar is one of the first three ingredients, it's a dessert. Here are two examples of how to use these simple rules at the point of contact.

1. Yogurt. A 20-ounce Coca-Cola has 27 grams of "total sugars." A standard 6-ounce Yoplait yogurt also has 27 grams of "total sugars." But yogurt's healthy, right? How much of those 27 grams is milk sugar (lactose, not harmful) and how much is added sugar (sucrose)? A Greek yogurt with no added sweeteners is 64 grams of total sugar per 24 ounces, or 16 grams per 6 ounces. That means that an individual Yoplait has 11 grams of added sugar. So when you consume a Yoplait, you're getting a yogurt plus 8 ounces of Coca-Cola.

2. Chocolate milk. Milk has calcium, phosphorus, and vitamin D, all
    necessary for growing children, and for adults to prevent osteopo-
    rosis. An 8-ounce carton of 1 percent milk has 130 calories and 15
    grams of "total sugars" (lactose). However, an 8-ounce carton of 1
    percent chocolate milk has 190 calories and 29 grams of "total
    sugars," including 14 grams of added sugar (HFCS). So chocolate
    milk is milk plus 10 ounces of Coca-Cola.

Yogurt and chocolate milk are perfect examples of how the food industry hides the sugar. The Nutrition Facts label lists "total sugars." If these
are from lactose (milk sugar) or from the sugar within the original fruit or
vegetable prior to packaging, they are not of concern. The only sugar that
you need be concerned about is the "added sugar," that which is specifically
added by the food industry for all the reasons just stated. The industry does
not have to report this number on the label, for "proprietary concerns" (see
chapter 16). But by checking the ingredient list and looking for the forty
names for added sugar, you can outsmart them.

Then we have the problem of juice. There's no added sugar, but there
is subtracted fiber, which makes the sugar in juice equivalent to sugar having been "added." This is one reason why the USDA Nutrition Facts food
label needs a complete overhaul (see chapter 21).

The goal of the supermarket exercise is to shift your food buying from
a high-fructose, high-trans-fat, low-fiber (i.e., processed) grocery basket to
a low-fructose, zero-trans-fat, high-fiber (natural) basket. The only rational
way is to buy real food in the first place. The meat, the dairy, the produce.
One of Michael Pollan's rules from his book *Food Rules* is "If your grandmother wouldn't recognize it as food, it isn't." Of course, your grandmother
might not recognize tempeh or tofu, miso or edamame—but someone's
grandmother would. I would also add that if the food has a company logo
you've heard of, it's processed. If you eat real food, your weight will take
care of itself, just as it did for the fifty thousand years since irrigation and
the taming of fire. We have no choice but to try to recreate the kind of food
supply our grandparents had, before the food processors tainted it. In the
UCSF WATCH Clinic, we provide the parents of our obese patients with a

shopping list where the foods are sorted by what they do to your insulin (table 17.2).

Table 17.2: A "Real" versus "Processed" Food Shopping List

The goal of obesity management is to keep your insulin down. This is a sample shopping list, based on four principles, to accomplish this goal:

1. Low sugar

2. High fiber

3. Low omega-6 fats

4. Low trans fats

Similar to the Traffic Light Diet, items listed as "green" can be eaten ad lib, those listed as "yellow" suggest mild caution (about three to five times per week), and those in "red" should be reserved for special occasions (about 1 to 2 times per week).

GREENS (unprocessed; ad lib)	YELLOWS (minimally processed; 3–5 times per week)	REDS (highly processed; 1 time per week)	LIMBO
INTACT WHOLE GRAINS			
High-fiber cereal (> 5 g fiber, < 3 g sugar)	Medium-fiber, medium-sugar cereal (> 3 g fiber, > 3 g sugar)	Refined grains (< 2 g fiber or >10 g sugar)	
Steel-cut (Irish) oatmeal: Bob's Red Mill (5 g fiber, 0 g sugar)	Rolled oats: Bob Red's Mill (4 g fiber, 1 g sugar)	Cream of Wheat	Diet anything
Shredded Wheat, no added sugar (7 g fiber, 1 g sugar)	Cheerios (3 g fiber, 1 g sugar)	Semolina	Sugar-free hot cocoa
Fiber One bran cereal (14 g fiber, 0 g sugar)	Nature's Path Organic Optimum Slim (11 g fiber, 10 g sugar)	White rice	Crystal Lite
Whole-grain bread (> 3 g fiber)	All Bran (10 g fiber, 6 g sugar)	Long-grain rice	Diet soda
German fitness bread	Kashi Go Lean (10 g fiber, 6 g sugar)	Arborio rice (risotto)	Propel
Coarse wheat kernel bread	Quaker High Fiber Instant Oatmeal (10 g fiber, 7 g sugar)	Jasmine rice	Diet Snapple

GREENS (unprocessed; ad lib)	YELLOWS (minimally processed; 3–5 times per week)	REDS (highly processed; 1 time per week)	LIMBO
Cracked wheat (Bulgur)	Kashi GOLEAN Crisp Toasted Berry Crumble (9 g fiber, 10 g sugar)	Bagels	Sugar-free flavored waters
Coarse barley kernel	Kashi GOLEAN Crunch! (8 g fiber, 12 g sugar)	White bread	
Coarse rye kernel (pumpernickel)	Raisin Bran (8 g fiber, 19 g sugar, partially from raisins)	Corn bread	
Whole-grain pumpernickel	Grape Nuts (7 g fiber, 5 g sugar)	Potato bread	
Whole grains	Go Raw Simple Granola (6 g fiber, 13 g sugar)	Rice bread	
Wild or brown rice	Frosted Mini Wheats (5 g fiber, 11 g sugar)	Croissants	
Whole amaranth	Ambrosial Granola (5 g fiber, 14 g sugar, partially from dried fruit)	Cinnamon roll	
Whole barley	Kix (3 g fiber, 3 g sugar)	Doughnuts	
Whole buckwheat	Total Whole Grain (3 g fiber, 5 g sugar)	Waffles	
Whole corn, including air-popped (unsweetened) popcorn	Laughing Giraffe Cherry Ginger Granola (3 g fiber, 8 g sugar)	Pancakes	
Whole millet	**Whole-grain products (pulverized whole grain)**	Couscous	
Whole oats	Whole-grain pastas	Basmati rice	
Whole quinoa	Protein-enriched pasta	Cake, brownies	
Whole rye	Whole-corn tortilla	Hamburger bun	
Whole sorghum	Whole-wheat tortilla	Hot dog bun	
Whole teff	**Breads (pulverized whole grain) (> 3 g fiber)**	Chips	
Whole triticale	Pita bread	Crackers	
Whole wheat—all whole wheat varieties	100 percent Whole Grain Natural Ovens	Pizza crust	

GREENS (unprocessed; ad lib)	YELLOWS (minimally processed; 3–5 times per week)	REDS (highly processed; 1 time per week)	LIMBO
Condiments	Oat Bran Bread	Rice Cakes	
All herbs	Healthy Choice Hearty 7 Grain®	Baguettes	
All spices	Buckwheat Bread	Rice Krispy®	
Earth Balance buttery spread	**Dairy**	Granola	
Homemade salad dressing	Sugar-free fruit flavored yogurt (a stretch)	Fruity Pebbles®	
Homemade barbecue sauce	**Meat (higher in omega-6, processed, higher in salt)**	**Proteins**	
Hummus	Commercial beef	Peanut butter and other commercial nut butters with more than two ingredients (Jif, Skippy)	
Lard	Ground beef	**Vegetables**	
Mustard	Hamburger	Baked potatoes	
Salsa	Baked beans	Tater tots	
Yogurt sauce	Chorizo	French fries	
Tabasco and other hot sauces (without sugar)	Sausage	Onion rings	
Vegetable Oils	Hot dog	Deep fried vegetables (breaded, fried in trans fat)	
Olive and canola oil are best for cooking, dipping, and salad dressings	Turkey bacon	**Fruits**	
Eggs	Turkey dog	Spreadable Fruit	
Eggs	Bacon	Fruit canned in syrup	
Egg Beaters	Salami, lunch meat	**Condiments**	

GREENS (unprocessed; ad lib)	YELLOWS (minimally processed; 3–5 times per week)	REDS (highly processed; 1 time per week)	LIMBO
Meat (low-omega-6, unprocessed)	**Fruits**	Sweet-and-sour sauce	
Grass-fed beef	Dried figs	BBQ sauce	
Wild fish	Dates	Ketchup	
Lamb	Banana chips	Teriyaki	
Turkey	Raisins	Ranch	
Free-range chicken	Unsweetened apple sauce	**Beverages**	
Nuts/Seeds	Dried pears	Soda	
Almonds	Craisins (dried cranberries)	Flavored milk	
Flaxseeds	Other dried fruits	Fruit juice—all, including organic, fresh squeezed, and commercial	
Macadamias	**Vegetables**	Chocolate rice milk	
Peanuts	Sweet corn	Chocolate soy milk	
Pecans	Red potatoes	Hot chocolate	
Pumpkin seeds	**Vegetable Oils and Fats**	Gatorade and other sport beverages	
Sunflower seeds	Safflower, corn, or soybean oil	Agua fresca	
Walnuts	Reduced-fat cream cheese	Lemonade	
Nut/seed butters: almond, cashew, macadamia, peanut hazelnut, and sunflower seed butter (all natural: made only of nuts/ seeds and salt)	Reduced-fat mayonnaise	Fruit smoothies	
Non-meat	**Condiments**	Sweetened iced tea	
Veggie/Garden Burger	Salt soy sauce	Sweetened coffee drinks	

GREENS (unprocessed; ad lib)	YELLOWS (minimally processed; 3–5 times per week)	REDS (highly processed; 1 time per week)	LIMBO
Boca Burger	Mayonnaise	Slurpies	
Tofu (made with calcium)	Cocktail sauce	Energy drinks	
Tempeh	Steak sauce	Vitamin water	
Dairy	Worcestershire sauce	Tomato juice	
Plain milk	Commercial salad dressing (made with canola or olive oil)	Vegetable juice	
Plain yogurt		**Condiments**	
String cheese		Commercial salad dressing (made with corn, soy, or safflower oil)	
Cottage cheese		Jam, jelly	
Mozzarella cheese		Honey	
Farmer's cheese		Maple syrup	
Cream cheese		Pancake syrup	
Jack cheese		Agave nectar	
Queso Fresco		Coconut oil	
Colby cheese		Palm oil, Palm kernel oil	
Cheddar cheese		Sugar	
Butter		Margarine (trans fats)	
Sour cream		Vegetable shortening (trans fats)	
Beans			
Adzuki beans, Anasazi beans, Black beans, Black-eyed peas, Edamame, Fava beans, Garbonzo beans (chickpeas), Kidney beans, Lentils, Lima beans			

GREENS (unprocessed; ad lib)	YELLOWS (minimally processed; 3–5 times per week)	REDS (highly processed; 1 time per week)	LIMBO
Fruits			
Apples, Apricots, Banana, Blueberries, Cantaloupe, Cherries, Grapes, Green bell peppers, Guava, Honey dew, Kiwi, Mandarin orange, Mango, Papaya, Peach, Pear, Pineapple, Plum, Raspberries, Star fruit, Strawberries, Watermelon, Any whole fruit (unprocessed)			
Vegetables			
Asparagus, Bean sprouts, Bell peppers (all colors), Bok choy, Broccoli, Carrots, Cauliflower, Cucumber, Eggplant, Green beans, Green peas, Lettuce, Mushroom, Onion, Peas, Peppers (all variety), Radish, Spaghetti squash, Spinach, Squash, Sweet potatoes, Tomato, Yams, Any whole vegetable (unprocessed)			
Beverages			
Water, Bottled water, Club soda, Sparkling water			
Plain milk (unflavored)			
Herbal and other teas (black and green) (unsweetened)			
Plain soy milk (fortified)	Flavored soy milk		

GREENS (unprocessed; ad lib)	YELLOWS (minimally processed; 3–5 times per week)	EDS (highly processed; 1 time per week)	LIMBO
Plain rice milk (fortified)	Flavored rice milk		
Coffee (black, no sweetener)	Sweetened coffee		

As real food costs more than processed food, many will view these recommendations as paternalistic and pejorative against the poor. However, only 19 percent of all money spent on food in the United States is for the food itself. The other 81 percent is for packaging and marketing. This is one hell of an upcharge, especially on the poor. If and when all America gets tired of paying it, maybe the food industry will rethink its strategies. (Occupy Nabisco, anyone?) In the meantime, they're going to ride this gravy train.

How to Eat Without Cooking

Not everyone can, has time to, wants to, or knows how to cook. While these people are at a minor disadvantage in eating real food, it's not impossible. The first rule is, stay out of fast food restaurants at all costs. No good can come of them. Beware packaged products, even those claiming to be organic. Many of them contain the same amount of sugar as their commercial counterparts. If you're buying a dish at a coffee shop or diner, make sure it has something green in it. Second, don't buy anything you can eat while standing up, because then you're not thinking about your food, and you're likely using your hands (which means more processed carbohydrates), not utensils. Sit down, enjoy it, make it a meal. Third, make sure it has some sort of protein—anything from sliced turkey to natural peanut butter is okay, just don't go for a baked good, which is just fat, carbohydrates, and sugar. Lastly, no smoothies or Frappuccinos™!

How to Survive a Restaurant

This chapter is about controlling your food environment. Restaurants are the ultimate loss of control. You have no control over what goes into the food, portion sizes, how quickly the food arrives, or whether there are bread or tortilla chips placed on the table before the meal. Plus, you must solve the immediate intellectual/emotional dilemma of volume versus taste versus price. No wonder buffets are so popular. So, does this mean you can never go to a restaurant again?

Portion sizes served at fast food restaurants have increased significantly since the 1970s. Sodas have increased by 49 calories, French fries by 68 calories, and hamburgers by 97 calories. Frequent fast food eaters consume more calories per day on average than non- or infrequent fast food eaters. Pricing and packaging encourage larger portions. In an experimental restaurant setting, customers who were served a larger portion ate 43 percent more. Children who eat at fast food restaurants twice a week increase their obesity risk by 60 percent, and those who frequent one three times a week, 300 percent.[26] There is a wide discrepancy between the number of calories customers expect to find in a fast food meal and the number they actually consume.[27] In addition, customers overestimate the healthfulness of fast food items that carry health claims. While salads and apple dippers are on the McDonald's top-ten list along with the Big Mac and French fries, most customers are not able to accurately assess the true caloric value of these so-called "healthy" options. Lastly, even when they rate a serving as too large, people will finish a larger portion merely because they've already paid for it.[28] Even having eaten more than they wanted, customers still see these "extra-value" meals as a good deal.

The rules for dealing with restaurants are very simple.

1. If the food comes in a wrapper, the wrapper has more health benefits than the food. Fast food restaurants are the antithesis of real food.
2. Whatever you do, don't order soda.
3. Ask the server not to put bread and chips on the table.

4. If you've already had dessert this week, don't make this your second.

So What's the Answer?

Do we need to avoid restaurants and supermarkets like the plague? Do we need to eat what our ancestors did or eschew all carbs? I would propose that all we need to do is eat "safe carbs." That means low sugar to prevent insulin resistance, and high fiber to reduce flux to the liver and prevent insulin hypersecretion. And while we're at it, eat "safe fat," that is, real fat rather than synthetic fat (such as trans fats, which can't be metabolized). Michael Pollan, in his *New York Times* article "Unhappy Meals," exhorts us to "Eat food. Not too much. Mostly plants." That's seven words; I'll reduce it to three: *eat real food.* The "not too much" will take care of itself. And the "mostly plants" isn't a worry if you eat the plants as they came out of the ground, or the animals who ate the food that came out of the ground—because they ate plants. The point missing in the various diet plans just explained is that all real food is inherently good. It's what we *do* to the food that is bad. Keep the food intact—you can steam, boil, or grill it. Food processing is the Mr. Hyde of this obesity pandemic. And the way to reverse it is to do the opposite.

Of course, this means major changes in the ways that both we and the food industry do business. But remember the early 1980s. The food industry had to overhaul its entire operation to adhere to the low-fat guidelines. It can do it again. One food industry executive told me, "We can change, with two provisos. We won't go it alone"—meaning the rest of the industry will need to follow suit—"and we can't lose money." Well, today, both of those are nonstarters. No doubt such changes would affect food prices. But it doesn't mean that everyone will have to pay more at the store. It all depends on how the U.S. government chooses to respond (see chapters 21 and 22). The battle against obesity must be waged on two fronts: at the individual level and at the public health level. Until the food industry, the grocery industry, and the restaurant industry realize that it is not in their best interest to provide our current processed food choices, don't expect our global food environment to improve anytime soon. Educating yourself as to what's in your food and what it does to you is half the battle to control your and your children's personal food environment. Educating government to improve everyone's food environment will be covered in detail in chapters 20–22.

Chapter 18

Altering Your Hormonal Environment

———————•———————

DeShawn is an eight-year-old African American boy who comes to clinic weighing 110 pounds and has a BMI of 35. He was referred due to an orthopedic condition in which both hips slipped out of their joints, limiting his motion and his ability to exercise. DeShawn is obstinate, confrontational, and doing poorly in school. His mother, while friendly and seemingly compliant, is also obese and very defensive. She tells us at each visit that she is doing exactly what we advise, ridding the house of sugared beverages, eating real food, and waiting twenty minutes for second portions. But at each clinic visit, DeShawn continues to show a gain in weight. Within three years, his weight is up to 255 pounds, and he has a BMI of 50. He develops obstructive sleep apnea, a potentially fatal illness, necessitating a call to Child Protective Services in an attempt to save his life. It is the thought of losing her son that forces the mother to face up to her own sugar addiction. She rids the house of the sodas that populated it, and she and De-Shawn both get psychiatric therapy. Within a year, each has lost 60 pounds, and DeShawn is conversant, pleasant, confident, and doing much better in school.

No doubt some of you will read this chapter and say, "What planet is this dude from? He talks about altering the 'hormonal environment,' but what he's really talking about is altering behavior. I could have gotten this out of any other self-help book." Au contraire, mon frère. We, both individually and as a society, need to do something differently to fix this pandemic. Clearly something needs to change. But change behavior? If you try to modify behavior you're doomed to failure, as evidenced by the sixty million diet recidivists nationwide. Indeed, when it comes to obesity, parents are incompetent at altering their children's behavior.[1] Most of the world views the word *behavior* as meaning the actions we choose to do or not through "free will." However, the dictionary definition of behavior is: "a stereotyped motor response to a physiological stimulus." The operative word here is *physiological*.

Felix Kreier in Amsterdam argues that "behavior" is the sum output of the genetic, hormonal, and biochemical inputs to the central nervous system that create specific drives.[2] What we call "behavior" is actually the cognitive inhibition on those biochemical drives. Yes, you can choose to ignore your cravings and skip the cookie. But can you really keep this up 24/7/365, when a hormone or a neurotransmitter is telling you to act and when the signal gets stronger with time? This isn't just thinking in the abstract; it has real practical applications. Every human behavior requires hormonal signals for expression (sexual behavior: androgen, estrogen; parental behavior: oxytocin). These behaviors truly are innate; they are the product of our biochemistry, which has developed evolutionarily for our survival. How else would parents not abandon their screaming two-year-old? Their hormones make them protective and form an immutable bond with their offspring. In one generation, our sugar glut has tweaked related hormones and neural pathways to our detriment. Of course, there are exceptions to this rule. But if the majority of us were able consistently to ignore our physiologic responses screaming for that doughnut, there wouldn't be a need for this book. Your body will always work against you, and you're doomed to fail.

The Way We Were

In trying to make sense of how all this works (or should I say *used to work*), I offer the insights of Markus Stoffel of the University of Zurich. He recounted his childhood: He ate lunch at noon, would get out of school at three, and then rush straight to the playground. For three hours, he and his classmates would play their hearts out and drink water from the school fountain. At 6:00 p.m. they'd return to their homes famished. "That six-hour interval of no food, only water, and vigorous activity was absolutely essential . . . to keep our livers happy, refreshed, and insulin sensitive, so the next day we could go at it all over again."

Forty years ago, soda was a treat and available only in 12-ounce cans. With the proliferation of the 2-liter soda bottle (patented by DuPont in 1973) and the Big Gulp, we, like DeShawn, now chug sugar as if it were going out of style. Parents work two jobs and don't have time to cook meals; kids are more stressed; playgrounds have disappeared due to housing and fear of crime, P.E. and sports have been slashed due to budget cuts. Our hormones worked in our previous environment of thirty years ago. They can still work, just not in the altered environment we have created for ourselves. And the sooner we realize what we've done to ourselves and to our children in the name of "progress," the sooner we can unravel it. Because, thus far, finding methods to adapt to our new environment has proven useless—witness the inefficacy of the "obesity profiteers." Face it: we're stuck with our hormones and our biochemistry. Many suffer from functional hormonal problems in one of the brain's eating pathways—hunger (chapter 4), reward (chapter 5), stress (chapter 6), or a combination of these three.

For 50–60 percent of the obese population, the following interventions should do the trick. For the rest of you, these interventions will be necessary, but likely not sufficient. More drastic measures will be required (see chapter 19). To dig ourselves out of this mess we need to fix the hormones to fix the behavior, and ultimately to fix our health. And to do so, we need to fix our environment.

Making Hormones Work for You

The roles of specific hormones in weight gain and metabolic dysfunction were elaborated in chapters 4–9. The goal of obesity management is to reverse the hormonal dysfunction by accomplishing the following:

1. Get the insulin down—to reduce your body fat and improve leptin resistance.
2. Get the ghrelin down—to reduce hunger.
3. Get the PYY up—to hasten satiety (the feeling of being full).
4. Get the cortisol down—to reduce perceived stress and hunger, and reduce deposition of energy into visceral fat.

1. Get the Insulin Down: Eat Fiber, Reduce Sugar, Exercise

For almost everyone, reducing insulin is the linchpin to success. Less insulin means less shunting of energy to fat cells, improved leptin sensitivity, and a lower appetite. It also means more energy available to muscles, which improves metabolic health and quality of life. How to get insulin down? That means reducing insulin release or improving insulin sensitivity, or both.

The best way to reduce insulin release is to limit the exposure of the pancreas to the agent that drives insulin up, which is glucose. This means cutting back on refined carbohydrates. Improving insulin sensitivity means improving hepatic, or muscle, insulin sensitivity, or both. And each one is accomplished differently. Improving hepatic insulin sensitivity means limiting the production of liver fat, which requires limiting your liver's exposure to fat and carbohydrates together (this is why most popular diets work, see chapter 17). The best way to do this is to reduce your sugar consumption, since this is always fat and carbohydrates combined. The easiest means of accomplishing this feat is to remove sugared beverages from your house: soda, juice, Vitamin Water, all of it. Stick with water and milk. A sugar-addicted parent (see chapter 5), similar to one who is drug addicted, will act as an "enabler," "co-dependent," or "apologist" for her child. The job of the parent is to convert the house from a minefield into a safe house for the child.

Another way to lower your insulin is to eat more fiber, which reduces flux to the liver and the insulin response (see chapter 12). Opt for brown foods: beans, lentils, whole grains, nuts, and other legumes. And eat the real stuff: the whole fruits and vegetables rather than their processed or juiced derivatives. White food—bread, rice, pasta, potatoes—means the fiber is gone (or, in the case of potatoes, was never there in the first place).

Finally, improving muscle insulin sensitivity is very simple—only exercise will do it, because once muscle fat is stored, the only way to get rid of it is to burn it off. Plus, exercise will burn off liver fat as well.

2. Get the Ghrelin Down: Eat Breakfast with Protein, Stop Nighttime Bingeing, and Sleep More

Reducing ghrelin, the hunger hormone (see chapters 6 and 11), will diminish total food intake at any given meal. And the best way to do so is to eat breakfast. If you don't eat breakfast, you don't ratchet up your thermic effect of food (see chapter 13), ghrelin levels keep rising as the morning drags on, and you will eat more at lunch, dinner, and into the evening. Eating breakfast is part of the equation, but what you eat makes a huge difference. A high-protein load has been shown to reduce ghrelin more than a meal high in fat or carbohydrates,[3] so you will burn more just sitting. Plus protein has a higher thermic effect, meaning it costs double the energy to metabolize protein versus carbohydrates. Plus protein doesn't generate nearly as high an insulin response as do carbohydrates, and doesn't lead to your blood glucose crashing down, which makes you hungry sooner. Bring on the bacon and eggs.

Some people with very severe insulin resistance, caused by overconsumption of sugar, are enormously hungry—so hungry that standard mealtime changes won't cut it. The hallmark of this pattern is nighttime bingeing.[4] When these patients awaken, they are not hungry and usually go without breakfast (which is a warning sign for big indiscretions later in the day). Indeed, they invariably eat before bed; some of them even awaken from sleep to eat. Eating after dinnertime is problematic for everyone, because any energy consumed that late will have no chance to be burned. It will find its way either to the fat tissue or to the liver, making the patient even more insulin resistant. Some of these patients also have obstructive sleep apnea, and virtually all of them have metabolic syndrome. They are enormously fatigued and can't find the ability to exercise, due to both the excess insulin and the lack of sleep.

In order to improve their leptin resistance, which means improving their insulin resistance, they must break this vicious cycle of nighttime eating and energy storage. The only hope these patients have is to readjust their mealtimes. This means eating a sensible breakfast and lunch with no snacks added, and dinner must consistently occur a good four hours before bedtime. Any late dalliances with food will only make matters worse. These patients must also get consistent sleep, which can be very difficult due to problems in their airways while sleeping (called obstructive sleep apnea). Patients who snore (and in this category they all do) may need to see their doctor to get a Bilevel Positive Airway Pressure (BiPAP) machine to hold their airway open while sleeping. Some patients may need a tonsillectomy and adenoidectomy to create a larger airway for better sleep.

3. Get the PYY Up: Eat Appropriate Portions, Wait Twenty Minutes for Seconds, Eat Fiber

A kid eats a whole plate of food and says to her mother, "I'm still hungry." Mom doesn't want her kid to starve, certainly doesn't want any whining, and serves up another portion. You parents out there, how many times has this happened to you? Every day? Every meal? For adults, why do you devour a second hamburger immediately after scarfing down the first? There is a huge difference between the phenomenon of satiety versus the phenomenon of lack of hunger (see chapter 12). Putting food in the stomach lowers your ghrelin, but that doesn't stop you from eating more. The signal for satiety—the switch that turns off the meal—is peptide $YY_{(3-36)}$. Between the stomach and the PYY cells are twenty-two feet of intestine. It takes time for the food to get there. Give it a chance. The Japanese have a saying, "Eat until you are 80 percent full." This is very difficult to do in America. The key is to wait twenty minutes for second portions. Also, make sure your first portion is an appropriate size—even if you don't go back for seconds, you're going to do damage if you've supersized your meal. The best way to get your PYY up is to make the food move through the intestine faster, and that's the job of fiber (see chapter 12). And the best way to get fiber is to eat real food.

4. Get the Cortisol Down: Exercise

Now here's the hard one. Cortisol is your short-term friend and your long-term enemy. Keeping cortisol low, which means keeping stress down, is virtually impossible. There are more stressors today than ever before, and no natural way to deal with them. Our ancestors may have run away from the attacking lion, but it is considered poor form to bolt full speed from your yelling boss. Stress-induced eating may be one of the toughest challenges to overcome. First, because it's not the stress, it's the *response to stress* that matters (see chapter 6). This may be either genetically or prenatally determined (see chapter 7), and unlikely to respond to simple willpower. Second, since excess cortisol drives visceral fat, insulin resistance, and further food intake, it's the triple whammy for metabolic syndrome. Finally, cortisol alters the output of the amygdala in a positive feedback, or vicious cycle, manner, so that more cortisol results in more amygdala activation, resulting in more cortisol the next time, and so on. Since nobody's stress is going away in this lifetime, the overeating won't go away either. If you've got poor coping mechanisms and everything in life is chaotic, it's pretty hard to ignore your troubles, and they tend to multiply.

There is one simple, cheap, and effective way to reduce your cortisol: exercise. Although exercise raises your cortisol while you're doing it (to mobilize glucose and free fatty acids for energy), it reduces your cortisol levels for the rest of the day. It burns off fat in your muscles to improve muscle insulin sensitivity, and in your liver to improve hepatic insulin sensitivity. In our clinic, the rule is to buy your screen time with activity. Every hour of TV or computer games means an hour of playing sports. This is the hardest for families to do, because parents tend to use the TV as a babysitter, and modern children tend to prefer playing sports with a joystick.

Many parents start dreaming about what college their child will attend before the kid is out of the womb. Your children feel that stress—which affects their mood, their actions, and their studies. The pressure on children today is enormous. Where can they find the time for everything? Here's perhaps the most important idea in this book for raising children. If your child lays off the soft drinks and exercises, he will *create time*. If he exercises vigorously for one hour, his five hours of homework will take only four hours because he will be more focused and efficient. He will have created time. There are numerous studies from around the country documenting that increasing exercise improves kids' school performance and behavior. Parents, creating time is what life is all about in the twenty-first century. You can't increase the number of hours in the day, but you can increase your child's productivity.

Sadly, your kids' school doesn't get it. They're saying, "We have to teach to the test, otherwise No Child Left Behind will pull our funding." Teachers, here's what you need to know: No Child Left Behind is really No Child Moving Forward and No Teacher Left Standing. Teachers, exercise your kids during the school day. Lose forty-five minutes from the daily schedule and devote it to real huffy-puffy, sweaty exercise. The kids will do better in school and exhibit better behavior.

The Way We Need to Be

Processed food altered our current environment. All the pieces are available for us to retool. For example, how about crockpot dinners made that morning? Salads don't need cooking—just be careful about the ingredients in the processed dressings. Kids need to bring lunch from home and not purchased at school, where, with a few notable exceptions, the food is highly processed, sugar-laden, frozen (so, it contains no fiber), shipped cross-country, and just plain nasty. Like DeShawn's mother, take the soda out of the house. Try to ensure that your child doesn't eat the home *and* school lunch or trade it with a classmate. Talk to your school principal about the food served at school; the school can do better. Make sure the convenience food trucks don't line up outside the school waiting for kids to exit with dollars in their fists. If your kid is old enough, how about having her cook for the family? She needs to learn sometime, or in college the freshman 50 will no doubt replace the freshman 15. Of course, these changes are applicable only to the middle and upper classes of society. The poor still do not have access to healthy foods or areas in which to exercise. This is one of the many reasons that public health solutions are also necessary (see chapters 20–22).

It's the Hormones, Stupid . . .

There are two ways to look at how our environment relates to obesity. The first one says that genes and behavior interact to drive weight gain. But both genes and behavior are unalterable; so in this paradigm, all is lost. The second says that behavior is the output of hormones (see chapter 4) and hormones are responsive to the environment. Obesity is a hormonal problem, and hormones are alterable, so in hormones there is hope. In this chapter, I've provided the rationale and methods to alter the environment, for even the most recalcitrant of patients. But that doesn't mean it will work. The precepts will work for 60–70 percent of the obese population. Sadly, genetics, epigenetics, developmental programming, and environmental obesogens can overwhelm any environmental alteration. Sometimes medicine and surgery are necessary.

Chapter 19

Last Resorts: When Altering
Your Environment Isn't Enough

———————•———————

Jared is a fifteen-year-old who has been obese his whole life. He is very self-aware and knows the repercussions, both medically and socially. We test him for genetic mutations, and nothing turns up. His oral glucose tolerance test exhibits massive insulin release, but no insulin resistance. We place him on octreotide, which stabilizes his weight for a total of ten months; but then his weight continues to increase. Other medicines are of no use. In his senior year of high school, he undergoes a laparoscopic adjustable gastric band (LAGB) procedure. Over the next year, his appetite abates, his weight reduces from 366 to 222 pounds. His mother reports, "We just went out to dinner, and I overheard someone at the next table say, 'What a good-looking family,' and I thanked God and started to cry."

Obesity is not a behavior. It is not even a disease (as that would assume a common pathophysiology). Indeed, obesity is a phenotype (a composite trait) of many different pathologies. Remember, there are three different organ systems that could be dysfunctional—the brain (see chapters 4–6); the fat (see chapters 7–9); or the hormones that affect the brain or the fat (see chapter 18). Obesity was, is, and will be, forever. But it need not exist at this frequency. The problems of hunger (hypothalamic dysfunction), reward (nucleus accumbens dysfunction), or stress (amygdala dysfunction) can overwhelm just about anyone. And if you create extra fat cells along the way (e.g., steroid use for cancer therapy, or extra insulin before birth due to the mother's prenatal diet or her gestational diabetes), those cells aren't going to give up their energy without a fight. Alterations in the food and hormonal environments will work for 50–60 percent of the population, but there will still be people who can't overcome those biochemical forces. To the best of our ability, we need to determine the individual basis for the obesity to best treat its underlying causes. Otherwise, we are fighting the wrong problem. The key to successful therapy in these patients is accurate diagnosis. Unfortunately, our diagnostic armamentarium is not yet fully developed, so matching treatment to diagnosis remains uncertain.

There is not, and never will be, a magic bullet for obesity or metabolic syndrome, especially if you consume four sodas a day. This chapter is written with the working assumption that a formal six-to-twelve-month period of food and hormonal environmental alteration—including psychodynamic, cognitive, and/or family therapy where necessary—has been attempted, and has not been effective. What then? It's time to move to the bigger guns.

Drilling Down Through the Fat: Laboratory Tests and Your Health

Chapter 8 reviewed methods for ascertaining your level of visceral fat. Every other method to assess your metabolic risk is relatively expensive and requires blood drawing, specialized equipment, and/or professional data analysis. These tests and their analysis should be left to your physician. But you should know what they mean, as they are important for gauging your health.

The Lipid Conundrum

Virtually everyone in America now gets a fasting lipid profile (aka cholesterol test) to assess their risk for heart disease. But there's a lot more to the lipid profile than meets the eye (see chapter 10), and this field is continually evolving. In the 1970s, scientists determined that LDL (low-density lipo-

proteins) were the bad type of cholesterol, whereas HDL (high-density lipoproteins) were beneficial. In the early 2000s, we learned that the
triglyceride (TG) level also correlated with heart disease risk, especially in
light of the obesity pandemic. The TG-to-HDL ratio is a surrogate marker
of oxidized LDL (the LDL that lines arteries), insulin resistance, and metabolic syndrome. When you get a fasting lipid profile, your doctor needs to
look at *all* the lipid fractions, as they cannot be viewed in isolation.

Alanine Aminotranferase (ALT)

Diagnosing metabolic syndrome is all about assessing the fat in the liver.[1]
While not specific for liver fat accumulation, the liver enzyme ALT is easy
to assess and is a good predictor of future diabetes.[2] Most doctors get nervous with an ALT above 40, but recent data argue that even an ALT of 25
predicts liver fat.

Fasting Insulin, Glucose, and Hemoglobin A_{1c}

Every doctor gets a fasting glucose on his adult patients, looking for type 2
diabetes. This parameter is the very last one to change; by the time it has
gone south, metabolic syndrome is in full force, and there are no options
for prevention anymore. The body will do everything it can to maintain the
serum glucose in the normal range, including increasing the insulin. (That's
insulin resistance!) So the way to interpret a fasting glucose is by getting a
simultaneous fasting insulin level, which tells you how hard the pancreas is
working. However, a fasting insulin will tell you only about insulin resistance. It won't tell you about excessive pancreatic insulin secretion.

In our clinic, we assume insulin resistance when we see a patient for
the first time, because it is so common. If the patient responds to an environmental intervention (see chapter 18), there is no further need for testing. If she doesn't, we use an oral glucose tolerance test to see if she releases
too much insulin[3] (see chapter 4), and then determine the best course of
therapy to lower insulin release.

Doctors have started to screen patients with hemoglobin A_{1c} (HbA_{1c}),
the blood test that assesses glucose control over the preceding three months

and is used to monitor diabetic patients. By everyone's estimation, under 5.5 percent is normal, over 6.5 percent is diabetes, while 6.0–6.5 percent requires a glucose tolerance test to determine if diabetes is present.[4]

Inflammation Markers

Metabolic syndrome is also about inflammation and cell damage. All these tests (such as high-sensitivity C-reactive protein) are very expensive, none is paid for by standard commercial insurance, and none has been shown to predict with precision the timing of a heart attack or stroke. Thus, while they show promise, all tests remain subjects of research and have not yet been adopted clinically.

Seeing Is Believing: Imaging Studies

When it comes to obesity, a picture truly is worth a thousand words. Is there any way to tell what your belly and your liver are up to? Yes, but they are all expensive, research-based, and not likely to be readily available soon. Liver ultrasounds have a high specificity for detecting fatty liver (meaning when it's there, you can see it), but the sensitivity is relatively low (meaning that you can think it's there, but it's not). Another test is called dual emission X-ray absorpiometry (DEXA). While fat tissue can very easily and nicely be quantified, it's impossible to tell what type it is (subcutaneous, visceral, or liver), so such a measure is of limited use. Two more methods are CT and MRI of the abdomen, which can differentiate the different storehouses of fat. Both MRI and CT cost more than $1,000 a pop and are not covered by insurance, which puts them out of the reach of most patients.

Once you know whether you're fat or sick or both, and once your doctor has ruled out specific genetic or biochemical abnormalities, you and your doctor can make a conscious decision as to the most appropriate mode of therapy, and how best to monitor your progress.

The Obesity Drug Pipeline—a Trickle, Not a Gusher

Sadly, drug therapy for obesity has hit the skids. It seems incredible that in the face of the relative lack of efficacy of lifestyle interventions, the ever-expanding knowledge of the physiology of energy balance, and a veritable gold mine for successful candidates, most pharmaceutical companies have closed their obesity research programs.

A new anticancer therapy that can show an increase in survival for four extra months can get FDA approval despite severe side effects, yet the bar has been set so high on obesity drugs that any that demonstrate even the slightest toxicity are doomed to failure. The FDA is tasked to do a cost-benefit analysis on every new drug. Are the potential side effects worth the risk? FDA commissioner Margaret Hamburg believes that obesity is about "making healthy choices," therefore, why would you need drugs? There are numerous medications for the diseases within metabolic syndrome, but virtually none targeting patients before these illnesses develop. The FDA has recently withdrawn three medications (ephedrine, sibutramine, and phenyl-propanolamine) due to concerns over potential toxicity. Only orlistat (Xeni-cal or its over-the-counter version, Alli) is still with us. Its long-term benefits are questionable, it has adverse effects galore, and is in a fight for its life over allegations of possible liver toxicity. The FDA recently voted down three combination drugs (although one of these, phentermine-topiramate, or Qsymia, made it through on the second try in 2012). And they just gave the go-ahead to lorcaserin in July 2012.

What's Left of Pharmacotherapy—Last Drug Standing?

This leaves very few medications to talk about. Furthermore, obesity drugs don't have a great track record. Energy balance is so crucial to survival that we want to hold on to our fat at any cost. Every obesity drug works for about four months, and then that negative plateau kicks in (see chapter 4). Every drug has side effects, some of them serious. Each drug is tested in combination with a low-calorie diet, therefore every drug must currently be considered an adjunct to standard environmental modification, which is not the way people use them in real life. You have to do the right thing anyway. Obesity drugs work on different aspects of energy balance. Currently, the approaches are: reducing calories eaten (phentermine), reducing energy absorbed (orlistat), increasing energy expended (nothing left here), and improving either insulin resistance (metformin) or suppression of insulin release (a low-carb diet).

While many new drugs are currently under study, and many of them are attempts at targeted therapy, proof of safety and efficacy are hard to come by. One reason is that obesity is not one disease but many, so each drug will work only in a percentage of people. Another reason is that the mechanisms to maintain your weight are redundant and strong, so treating one pathway is often not enough. Many experts have abandoned the idea of a big blockbuster agent that will "cure" obesity,[5] and have instead started advocating combination drugs that target different parts of the energy balance pathway. But that means drug companies would have to work together, which is like expecting Apple to love Microsoft. And that means no home runs, only the occasional single. Just as in baseball, don't expect the pharmaceutical houses to invest the bankroll for a singles hitter.

Bariatric Surgery—Not a "Magic Scalpel"

In adults with comorbidities and in adolescents with extreme and life-threatening obesity, surgical therapy may be necessary. Bariatric surgery can not only promote weight loss, but also reverse type 2 diabetes in up to 50 percent of patients, and might help you live longer.[6] Yet it is virtually impossible to perform randomized controlled trials of bariatric surgery due to ethical concerns; you can't do a sham surgery on people. And no studies take the causes or mechanisms of the obesity into account. So the efficacy of targeting any approach to any given patient will continue to be suspect.

Bariatric surgery is most effective in preventing the development of the various comorbidities associated with obesity before they take hold, such as diabetes and obstructive sleep apnea. By the time you have developed these disorders, surgery may improve them but will likely not reverse their presence. However, many insurance companies will not approve this procedure until you qualify with one of these life-threatening diseases.

Also, if you wait until you are severely obese (more than 450 pounds), you are unable to have the surgery anyway, as you cannot fit in an MRI scanner, which is needed to observe your post-op progress. A catch-22.

In adolescents, performing surgery early in the game (only among the severely obese) will likely add years to their lives. They may even be spared the ravages of metabolic syndrome. However, the insurance company will opt to wait as long as possible, when the patient is no longer covered under his parents' insurance. Therefore, guidance is needed to determine the ideal circumstances when the balance of risk versus benefit favors health improvement and reversion of complications, yet with the lowest risk of morbidity and mortality.

Surgical outcomes in adults vary between surgeons and institutions. The only method to validate and refine the use of these procedures comes from following patients carefully and long term,[7] which is of no use to the patients undergoing surgery today. It is absolutely essential that bariatric surgery be performed in regionalized academic centers with programs equipped to handle the data acquisition, long-term follow-up, and multidisciplinary nature of these difficult patients.[8] However, by restricting the number of sites, you limit the number of surgeries that can be performed, and access to them.

One of the biggest public misconceptions is that bariatric surgery consistently works in the long term. That's the party line toed by the media, the bariatric centers, celebrities such as Al Roker, Sharon Osbourne, and Star Jones, and the "cut-and-run" surgeons. But for how long? Virtually everyone loses weight for the first twelve months.[9] But the real story is told after the one-year breakpoint. Up to 33 percent of patients gain much if not all their weight back.[10] The stomach can easily restretch to accommodate excessive food intake. In many procedures, the stomach is reduced from the size of a baseball glove to that of a golf ball. The sensation of hunger is reduced, and the feeling of fullness is achieved after smaller portions are consumed. Great. But, as mentioned, many of the obese don't only eat when they are hungry. The underlying causes of the obesity—the "behaviors" of reward and stress (see chapters 5 and 6)—are not even remotely alleviated by these procedures, and not addressed by most patients or doctors. And the procedure doesn't prevent you from drinking your calories, which will bring you back to your initial weight even faster. These patients need long-term psychotherapy in addition to surgery. The point is that bariatric surgery is an adjunct to dietary and environmental change, not a "magic scalpel."

You Can Pay Me Now, or You Can Pay Me Later

Very few people can afford to have these procedures, as they can cost anywhere from $15,000 to $40,000 just for the surgery, let alone the pre-op evaluation, any complications, and the long-term follow-up. If Al Roker and Sharon Osbourne can get it, why can't you? Because your insurance company doesn't want to pay for it. Yet several cost-benefit analyses have been done that say that bariatric surgery increases both longevity and quality of life.[11] It actually reduces health-related costs, especially those associated with treating type 2 diabetes. And the strain on the medical system—by 2030 we will be taking care of a hundred million diabetics in the United States alone—might just ease slightly.

Bariatric Procedures

Bariatric procedures (colloquially referred to as "stomach stapling") can be divided into malabsorptive (food goes out in the stool), restrictive (food can't get into the stomach), and a combination of the two. Purely malabsorptive procedures (such as the duodenal switch and the jejuno-ileal bypass) have extremely high morbidity and mortality, and cannot be recommended. The Roux-en-Y gastric bypass (RYGB) is a combination procedure, which not only leads to extraordinary weight loss but can reverse type 2 diabetes as well.[12] The restrictive procedures reduce stomach volume to decrease the volume of food ingested. They include the Bioenteric Intragastric Balloon (BIB),[13] laparoscopic adjustable gastric band (LAGB),[14] and sleeve gastrectomy (SG).[15] Unfortunately, the general safety of these procedures correlates inversely with the degree of weight loss—the safer the procedure, the less weight lost—so there is no "favored" type.

Bariatric Surgery in Children

Unlike with adults, stricter and more conservative criteria must be applied to adolescents, since only 85 percent of obese adolescents will become obese adults; the slightly improved rate of lifestyle and pharmacotherapeutic efficacy versus that of adults; a longer time interval before comorbidities become life-threatening; and children's inability to give legal consent. For all these reasons, an expert panel with representation from the American Pediatric Surgical Association and the American Academy of Pediatrics has suggested that bariatric surgery for adolescents should be done only in institutions committed to long-term management of these patients,[16] and is justified in situations when obesity-related comorbid conditions (such as obstructive sleep apnea) threaten the child's health. While I must accede to this view, my personal feeling is that usually the horse is out of the barn by then. Waiting until a child is fully grown can mean many more pounds and much more comorbidity, which could be avoided by confronting the problem earlier. It is easier to stabilize weight gain than it is to induce weight loss. But the degree to which this surgery should be used as a solution will have to wait until we have further data.

Last Resorts versus First Passes

The fact that any of the medications or procedures in this chapter exist, let alone are common, speaks to the breakdown of our energy balance pathway and the alterations in our environment that have led to that breakdown. These last resorts are clearly necessary for the 5 percent of the population who have a biochemical abnormality, and who would have been obese ten, one hundred, or even a thousand years ago. But for the other 95 percent of people, of whom 60 percent are overweight or obese, and for the 40 percent of normal-weight people who have metabolic syndrome, do we have to jump to last resorts first? Do we have the money for last resorts for every obese patient in America? Clearly, something needs to happen on the first pass. And that's where public health comes in. Part 6 will make the argument that public health is our best and only chance worldwide to turn this juggernaut around.

PART VI

The Public Health Solution

Chapter 20

The "Nanny State":
Personal versus Societal Responsibility

———————•———————

"The proverb warns that, 'you should not bite the hand that feeds you.' But maybe you should—if it prevents you from feeding yourself."

—Thomas Szasz, psychiatrist and social critic, author of *The Myth of Mental Illness* (1960) and *The Manufacture of Madness: A Comparative Study of the Inquisition and the Mental Health Movement* (1970)

We live in a cop-out culture. We espouse personal liberty and responsibility. The American Dream tells us that any citizen can be president one day. Our libertarian leanings dictate that we are in control of ourselves and of our lives. Any challenge to our personal authority is unwanted, unwelcome, and considered un-American. Until the bottom drops out, and then we look for someone to blame, and demand increased regulation. Occupy Wall Street is a perfect example.

Personal Responsibility versus Public Health

Our libertarian philosophy says, "You, and only you, are in charge of your own health. Public health is the medical manifestation of the 'nanny state.'" Public health is concerned with the health of the entire community, not just the individual. It has been said that "health care is vital to all of us some of the time, but public health is vital to all of us all the time." How dare the school district demand that my children be immunized? How dare the airport official confiscate my pineapple at the Honolulu Airport? How dare the state check me for syphilis before I get married? Acute public health problems always occur to someone else. Someone else gets TB from bad hygiene. Someone else gets lockjaw from stepping on a rusty nail. It's your choice, right? Yet your opinion generally changes when you're the one who gets sick or it is your child who dies of Rubella because either he or his classmate went unvaccinated. And that's the paradox of public health; it's always somebody else's problem . . . until it's yours. Same with obesity.

If We're All Co-Opted, Who's the Nanny?

Ultimately, how well our society does in solving the obesity pandemic depends on its responses to the following questions. Which of the following is the fault of the individual? When a kid's brain thinks it's starving? When the American Academy of Pediatrics still recommends juice for toddlers, and the American College of Obstetrics and Gynecology still recommends juice for pregnant women? When the first ingredient in barbecue sauce is high-fructose corn syrup and when soda is cheaper than either milk or water? When high-fiber fresh produce is unavailable in poor neighborhoods due to lack of supermarkets and associated costs? When the local fast food restaurant is the only neighborhood venue that is clean and air-conditioned? When in order to meet the criteria for No Child Left Behind, and in the face of budget cuts, the school does away with P.E.? When children are not allowed out of the house to play, for fear of crime?

All health debacles were originally categorized as personal travails before they were declared public health issues. Cholera, tuberculosis, lead poisoning, vitamin deficiencies, pollution/asthma—these were all considered "personal responsibility" before the sheer magnitude of morbidity or mortality commanded governmental intervention. In each case, the science had to be elaborated before rational governmental policies could be designed and implemented. And in each case, politics initially stood in the way, on either economic or religious grounds. Vaccinations are important not only for the individual but also for the community as a whole. It's known as "herd immunity." As a result of regulations and sometimes forced vaccinations, we have nearly eradicated polio and other highly infectious diseases. Teen pregnancy was going up at an alarming rate in America from the 1960s through the 1980s. Similarly, HIV/AIDS ran rampant through the 1980s. Both were assumed to be matters of personal responsibility. It wasn't until Surgeon General C. Everett Koop convinced the nation that AIDS was a public health crisis on the basis of the science of HIV propagation, and needed to be responded to as such, that we started to see a decline in the prevalence of either one.

And then there are the chronic public health problems that transpire among the unsuspecting populace. Witness the increased incidence of cancer in the inhabitants of Love Canal. Or the epidemic of spina bifida in newborns as a result of their mothers being deficient in folic acid. Or the incidence of asthma in the survivors of the attacks on the World Trade Center on 9/11. Sometimes it requires public outcry to coerce the government into action—witness regulations on lead paint and the removal of asbestos.

And finally, there are the two biggest public health demons that now exist worldwide: tobacco and alcohol. Use of tobacco or alcohol is clearly a personal issue—except that it isn't. Tobacco and alcohol abuse elevate to public health status for two reasons: *your* smoking and drinking affect *me* (also known as externalities; see chapter 22), and tobacco and alcohol are both addictive substances. Addictive substances thwart all attempts at arguing solely for personal responsibility. Virtually every substance that activates the nucleus accumbens (e.g., cocaine, amphetamines, morphine, heroin, nicotine, alcohol) has required both a personal intervention—for lack of a better word, rehab—and some sort of public health intervention to control the environment, called laws. For instance, alcohol-control policies are in place in every country around the globe, along with an extensive body of evidence documenting strategic efficacy (see chapter 22). Tobacco-control policies have lagged behind, but they are catching up worldwide as well. Even Italy has recognized that the health care dollars saved by tobacco control more than justify the *stato di bambinaia*.

Do Nannies Know Best?

Within the last twenty years, the government has stepped in to curtail tobacco advertising targeted at youth. Camel has long since admitted that its
icon, Joe Camel, was designed to be "cool" to children and adolescents.
Recognizing that this was a public health issue, tobacco advertisements
were bannd from television and billboards near schools.

Which brings us to our food supply. I think we can all agree that the
global obesity pandemic is a monumental public health disaster. Although
most people are comfortable with food safety as a public health issue, many
critics warn that regulating food quality is the most egregious reach of the
"nanny state." But, in fact, the FDA was created to keep our food supply
safe. I would argue that food quality is equivalent to *long-term* food safety.
My daughter got *E. coli* from an undercooked hamburger at a Girl Scout
picnic in 2008. While *E. coli* will make you very sick, the probability is it
won't kill you. And it wouldn't cause the death of millions, because the FDA
would step in and recall the tainted product, as it did with tainted spinach
in 2010. Unfortunately, the FDA stands idly by while our current food supply is slowly poisoning the majority of the U.S. population.

Is Our Food Supply Tainted?

What if our breakfast cereal were laced with heroin by some unscrupulous
food company? Isn't it the role of government to protect us? If Coca-Cola
hadn't taken the cocaine out of its cola in 1903, the U.S. government certainly would have. And we have learned from tobacco documents how the
industry manipulated nicotine levels to increase the addictive potential of
cigarettes. One similarity in the industrialization of drugs of abuse versus
fast food is the addition of other compounds to increase saliency. For instance, menthol is frequently added to cigarettes. In 2011 the Tobacco
Products Scientific Advisory Committee of the FDA showed that "menthol
has cooling and anesthetic effects that reduce that harshness of cigarette
smoke," and that this effect "could facilitate initiation or early persistence of
smoking by youth."[1]

Similarly, food processors use additives to enhance flavor, color, texture, shelf life, and other attributes of palatability. For example, the presence of HFCS in fast food hamburger buns increases the sweet flavor and extends shelf life. Similarly, trans fats are superior for deep-frying (as with doughnuts and French fries) because they oxidize less readily than vegetable oils. In one study examining how fast food restaurants plan their menus, senior executives identified shelf life and spoilage as major obstacles to offering healthier items.[2] In the end, food processing results in combinations and concentrations of nutrients that are not present in nature, and that possess potential for abuse.

To the extent that sugar acts on the same reward pathways as drugs of abuse (see chapter 5) and poses the same harms to health, we must start wondering whether it should also be subject to public health controls. Yet in contrast to alcohol and tobacco, regulatory controls on sugar and sugar-containing processed foodstuffs are virtually nonexistent (see chapter 21).

Economic Freedom Doesn't Work with Addictive Substances

Economists (and food companies) routinely invoke the rule of the free market to govern the sales of food around the world. This makes perfect sense, except when it doesn't. Addictive substances don't follow the free market. As an example, in the midst of the economic recession and in the face of stiff competition from competitors, Starbucks raised its prices on coffee even though jet fuel prices took a nosedive. Apparently, spending six dollars a day on coffee is now common practice, just as George Carlin predicted.[3] Sugar is no different: its cost does not follow the free market. After all, would you really spend five dollars for a box of cereal or one dollar for a can of soda if it did? Despite the Great Recession, Americans have continued, if not increased, their consumption of addictive substances such as alcohol, tobacco, and chocolate. Coincidence?

We're Already Living in the Nanny State

The food industry currently has carte blanche over what can be put in a food and how it can be processed, packaged, and marketed. This has worked very well by increasing sales, decreasing depreciation, and expanding markets worldwide. The food industry has a vested interest in blocking any form of regulation, no matter the consequences on our public health. It has set up political action groups to help sway the populace into believing that any regulation is an affront to your liberty and an example of the "nanny state" in action. An example of such propaganda is the Center for Consumer Freedom (CCF), a nonprofit lobby group that serves as a front for the food industry. The purpose of CCF is to "defend the right of adults and parents to choose how they live their lives, what they eat and drink, how they manage their finances, and how they enjoy themselves." Their job is to convince you, the public, that you have the inalienable right to choose and eat any food product you wish, irrespective of its calorie content, sugar content, toxicity, abuse, or environmental impact.

That would be a great selling point if you actually had access and choice to *all* foods. But you don't. Unless you grow it yourself, you have only the access the food industry supplies to you. Barry Popkin of the University of North Carolina states that of the six hundred thousand food items for sale in the United States, 80 percent are laced with added sugar. Ninety percent of the food produced in the United States is sold to you by a total of *ten* conglomerates—Coca-Cola, ConAgra, Dole, General Mills, Hormel, Kraft, Nestle, Pepsico, Procter and Gamble, and Unilever. And the poor have only the foods they can get through SNAP and WIC, nearly all of which are processed and loaded with sugar for reduced depreciation. The point is, if you want to avoid sugar, you can't, because we already live in the nanny state. In fact, I would submit that by promoting the availability and consumption of real food, I am doing more to reverse the nanny state than any corporate entity, irrespective of advertising budgets or taglines; and than any government entity, irrespective of price controls or subsidies.

It's a War, and They're Winning

When it comes right down to it, it's really only about money—how to turn your money into their money. Figure 20.1 demonstrates the stock price of McDonald's, Coca-Cola, and PepsiCo as compared to the Standard and Poor 500 (S&P) as a percent change over the last five years. Despite the economic downturn that occurred in 2008, which has kept the stock market depressed, food-processing companies have consistently outperformed the S&P. Want to make money? Invest in a food company.

Personal Responsibility versus Public Funding for Health Care

Personal responsibility is a core American value. Personal responsibility and capitalism go hand in hand—take the risk, make the money. This allows the food industry to espouse their mantra: "Any food can be part of a balanced diet," including sugar. And since sugar is addictive, we'll eat it at

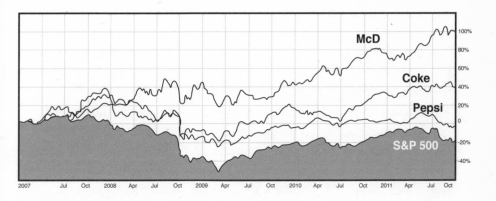

Fig. 20.1. Who's Winning the War? Changes in the stock price of McDonald's, Coca-Cola, and Pepsico for the years 2007–2011, in comparison with the S&P 500 Index. Despite the economic downturn of 2008, stock prices of McDonald's, Coca-Cola, Pepsico, and other food companies—ConAgra, General Mills, Hormel, Kraft, and Procter and Gamble not shown—all outstripped the S&P 500 over this time interval.

any concentration and at any cost. It allows the pharmaceutical industry a bigger market. It allows the propagation of the "obesity profiteers." When the government intervenes at all, it conveniently leaves itself out. Witness Michelle Obama's Let's Move! campaign, which says, focus on the individual, focus on the family, focus on the community. Missing from this equation are government and the food industry. It's a good show, gets a lot of airtime, and makes it look like something is happening—because it's deemed "personal responsibility." *Necessary, but not sufficient.* And nothing changes.

Forget the philosophical argument. Why should the government rethink obesity? Because it pays twice. First, it pays $20 billion for the annual corn and soybean subsidies, way more than for tobacco. Second, it pays for the emergency room visits for the strokes, heart attacks, and dialysis. A. B. Shaw, a British physician, once said, "Aortic valve operations on the elderly are very cost-effective if the result is death or cure instead of prolonged illness." If you can fix a chronic disease, it's worth the money to do it. But we can't cure cardiovascular disease, diabetes, cancer, kidney disease, or dementia. These diseases are eating away our health care dollars faster than we can print the money to pay for them.[4]

These are big numbers, and they're getting bigger every year. And this is happening to twenty- to forty-year-olds who will be sick for twenty to forty years. President Obama based the Patient Protection and Affordable Care Act (ACA, or "Obamacare") on the notion that there would be major cost savings in providing preventive services. If we continue to subsidize corn, promote processed food, and espouse personal responsibility for obesity, there won't be any prevention. Worker productivity will continue to decline, preventable chronic disease rates will continue to rise, and Medicare will be broke by the year 2024.[5] That's the outcome of "personal responsibility" with public funding. You can't have it both ways.

We really have only two choices. It's either personal responsibility all the way—if you get sick, you pay or you die. That's the Russian system. And of course it's done wonders for curbing their alcoholism, hasn't it? Or it's public health all the way—and we all get behind some societal interventions that can tame this beast.

The Nanny's Charges

Societal interventions can target either the affected individual or the entire population. There are strengths and limitations to both strategies, as listed in table 20.1.

Table 20.1: Strengths and Limitations of Personal versus Societal Interventions for Obesity

Strengths	Limitations
Personal interventions: Focus on the individual	
• Targets care only to the obese patient	• Patient is medicalized and demonized—"it's your fault"
• Limits money spent to those affected by obesity	• Offers no prevention for those who will be affected in the future—all those "flippers"(thin people who became fat along the way)
• Is easy to incorporate into medical care	• High costs and questions about feasibility
• Has clear and favorable risk-to-benefit ratio	• Emphasizes behavior modification, which has limited success in a "toxic environment"
	• Doesn't help thin people with metabolic disease
Societal interventions: Focus on the environment	
• Regulates quality of food nationally, improving health of everyone	• Must be acceptable to the general population; challenges the electability of politicians
• Changes food structure and availability	• Must be feasible; pushback expected from food companies and the addicted populace
	• Costs are prohibitive

While it might be more palatable to the populace to focus specifically on the obese, such across-the-board labeling may be too pejorative to be effective. Furthermore, don't forget that 20 percent of the obese population doesn't need targeted health care intervention, while 40 percent of normal-weight people need it, and won't get it. Lastly, altering one person's food environment is downright impossible. It's way easier to alter everyone's food environment at the same time. I offer the next two chapters as a smorgasbord of ideas to think about in order to help rescue our brethren and our economy before they both collapse under their own weight.

Chapter 21

What Hath Government Wrought?

———————•———————

**The Hyderabad Statement: "All significant public health
interventions involve and require the use of law."**

In 2000, the Memphis Area Society for Parenteral and Enteral Nutrition, with which I was affiliated, obtained an audience with the
Memphis Board of Aldermen. We discussed the increase in the obesity epidemic coincident with the transition of the lowest-income
neighborhood into a "food desert." The withdrawal of the only supermarket and the proliferation of fast food concessions were in part responsible for this change. We argued for zoning restrictions on the
density of fast food establishments in these neighborhoods. One of
the senior aldermen calmly asked the question "You want to take away
the single thing in these people's lives that gives them pleasure?"

I didn't have an answer for that question then and I'm not sure I have one
now. If the goal is short-term pleasure, the alderman is right. If the goal
is for business to make money, he is also right. But if the goal is health; happiness; medical, economic, and social justice; and overall societal benefit,
then his is just the type of thinking that prevents us from achieving it.

"Government Is Not the Solution to Our Problem, Government *Is* the Problem"

In no arena has President Reagan's signature quote been truer than in the government's passive role fomenting the obesity epidemic. Throughout our history, bills and programs designed and funded with the best of intentions have been adulterated and abused by multiple stakeholders, each with a hand out (see chapter 2), and with no interest in a mutually beneficial solution.

Joseph, Pharaoh, and the Farm Bill

Our nutritional crisis is the long-term result of the Farm Bill. The Farm Bill is one of the most complex and antiquated pieces of renewable legislation that Congress approves every five years. It was developed in the 1930s for two reasons: First, we had family farmers who were succumbing to a double whammy, the Depression and the Dust Bowl. Second, we had a hungry and destitute population. The country needed cheap calories, and that meant storable commodities: wheat, rice, soybeans, corn, grains you can put in silos or ship around the country without fear of spoilage. This happened in ancient Egypt when, in Genesis 41:33–36, Joseph told Pharaoh he would need to store grain in preparation for seven years of famine. Crops without a lot of water that don't shrivel up when you dry them. Not a green vegetable in the bunch.

The Farm Bill was developed with subsidies for all forms of storable carbohydrate. This produced a glut of high-glucose foodstuffs, which, over time, meant two things—we had to find new uses for them (e.g., ethanol for cars) and we had to get people to eat more of them. Here we find the basis for our current nutritional policy and the reason that grains have formed the basis of the USDA Food Pyramid for decades: an antiquated, unneeded policy that needs big-time reform, and one that rewards the richest 10 percent of farmers. But because the midwestern agricultural states maintain so much political clout, with two senators per state despite their sparse populations, tinkering with the Farm Bill remains political suicide. Try it at your own risk.

A recent report entitled "Apples to Twinkies: Comparing Federal Subsidies of Fresh Produce and Junk Food" documents a five-year allocation of $16.9 billion for corn and soy syrups and oils versus a total of $262 million for apples. At the individual level, that's $7.36 per year for junk food (worth nineteen Twinkies) and $0.11 per year for apples (worth a quarter of one apple),[1] or as Michael Pollan succinctly put it, "If you've got one dollar to spend on food, are you going to buy 1200 calories in potato chips or 200 calories in carrots?"

A total of $190 billion (two thirds) of the Farm Bill is used for nutrition programs, primarily for the indigent—such as SNAP, WIC, the Emergency Food Assistance Program, and the National School Lunch Program (NSLP). The goals for these programs are all the same: provide cheap nutrition with all the subsidized excess food. For instance, WIC was created to prevent "failure to thrive" in babies born to poor mothers. Unfortunately, the epidemic of obesity in poor children is the equal and opposite reaction. Until 2007, fruit juice was in the WIC portfolio, but fruit was not—because fruit juice was cheap and fruit was not. Indeed, frozen orange juice is traded on the commodities exchange, but fruit isn't. And even though fruit is now available through WIC, kids and mothers are still voting with their feet and choosing fruit juice anyway, for convenience and reward.

The final and most insidious reason is that badmouthing the food industry or the Farm Bill is the "third rail" of American politics. Because it's all about Iowa. Iowa is the first presidential contest for both parties. And that means no one wants to diss corn, or any corn-based product. In May 2011, I shared the dais at a Culinary Institute of America meeting with Sam Kass, of Michelle Obama's Childhood Obesity Task Force. Kass is not just any old chef. He is a very good-looking, smart, eloquent, and charismatic dude. I got twenty minutes alone with him, and he admitted to me that everyone in the White House, including the president, had read the *New York Times Magazine* article "Is Sugar Toxic?" (April 17, 2011), in which our UCSF research is featured. They wish me well—and they will do absolutely nothing to help. Not a plug, not a wink, not a nod. Nothing. Because they don't want the fight; this administration has enough enemies. I'm on my own, and you're on your own.

The FDA and the 1986 Fructose-GRAS Determination

Designation of a food additive as "generally regarded as safe" (GRAS) by the FDA allows food manufacturers to use any amount of it in food preparation without concern. Sugar was afforded GRAS status back in 1958, owing to its natural origin and long history of use, rather than to any science or toxicological analysis. In 1983 the FDA granted GRAS status to HFCS as well. Under pressure from a committee from the Federation of Experimental Biology, the FDA commissioned a "final" report on the effects of sugars on health. Led by Walter H. Glinsmann, a food scientist and FDA administrator (and now on the board of directors of the Corn Refiners Association—coincidence?), the authors of the 1986 report affirmed that "high fructose [corn] syrup is as safe for use in food as sucrose, corn syrup and invert sugar (the breakdown product of sucrose)."[2] The report also concluded that "fructose is a valuable, traditional source of food energy, and there is no basis for recommending increases or decreases in its use in the general food supply or in special dietary use products." In fact, the only problem sugar afforded humans was tooth decay, and that was easily solved by water fluoridation.

There are three problems with this determination. First, the data came way before the sugar glut. The report's correlations were based on the 1980s average sugar consumption of 40 pounds per person per year, which accounted for 200 calories per day, well within the American Heart Association upper-limit recommendations.[3] We're now at 130 pounds per person per year. Second, the authors of the report were looking at obesity, not metabolic syndrome—the term hadn't even been coined until 1988. And fructose does not specifically cause obesity; it turns obesity into metabolic syndrome. Lastly, like Ancel Keys (see chapter 10), they had no way to separate the effect of fat from the effect of sugar. In other words, they just plain missed the boat. Which is understandable, considering the science available at the time. But things have changed: obesity is rampant, and people are dying. Nonetheless, the FDA reaffirmed its stance in 1996 and again in 2004.[4] In response to our argument over the toxicity of sugar in the journal *Nature*,[5] an FDA spokesperson publicly stated that there are no plans to revisit this issue. Other countries have also turned a deaf ear to concerns about sugar. The European Food Safety Authority (EFSA) issued a statement in 2010 that it had found no scientific evidence to recommend a limit on the amount of sugar people should consume.[6]

Sugar Tariffs and Crony Capitalism

Sugar tariffs are the longest-running U.S. policy of all, dating back to 1789, when the First Congress imposed a tariff upon foreign sugar to raise revenue for the fledgling government. Since then, the sugar tariffs have expanded to increase competition with other subsidized countries, to provide protection for American jobs, and to make money for sugar czars to funnel back to politicians. Sugar is produced in 18 states, supports 146,000 U.S. jobs, and contributes $10 billion to the economy each year.

Due to the sugar tariffs, U.S. sugar prices currently are at or near record highs. Consumers on the world market pay $0.34 per pound for refined sugar, which is $0.20 less than Americans pay. While sugar tariffs generated $2.5 billion in 2009,[7] America's artificial price prop adds $1.4 billion to the shopping bills of U.S. consumers each year. All this has made a lot of people very wealthy. If these sugar tariffs actually reduced sugar consumption, I would be a proponent. But they don't. Despite the tariffs, the United States consumes more sugar per capita than any other country (see chapters 11 and 16). One reason is our addiction to sugar. The other is that the food industry has a very cheap alternative to sucrose in the form of HFCS.

The Executive Branch: Feeding the Food Industry

The executive branch has a vested interest in maintaining our current food structure and supply. To them, it's all about money and jobs. U.S. consumers spend approximately $1 trillion annually on food, which accounts for nearly 10 percent of the gross domestic product (GDP), and 6 percent of our exports revolve around food, accounting for another $56 billion. More than 16.5 million Americans are employed in the food industry,[8] and this number is not expected to decline over the next decade. The government will go to great lengths to keep us consuming at the same, if not increased, rates. And nearly all our consumption includes some sort of sugar. Yet the executive branch also doles out $147 billion annually in health care, most of it for chronic disease. It is in a no-win situation, and so the government tries to play both sides.

Sugar Extortion: The George W. Bush Administration versus the World Health Organization

In 2002, WHO and FAO convened a policy forum to address the role of nutrition in disease. They produced Technical Report Series (TRS) 916, entitled "Diet, Nutrition, and the Prevention of Chronic Diseases."[9] This document created a firestorm of controversy. Even a decade prior, no fewer than twenty-three countries had identified sugar as a major contributor to chronic disease. TRS 916 called for limiting added sugar to less than 10 percent of the total calories in the diet. Clearly, this could not stand. Dr. Riaz Khan, director of the World Sugar Research Organization, countered, "The concept of good food and bad food lacks scientific credibility . . . Every food can make a valuable contribution to diet and diet variety; it is getting the balance right that is the key."

Time for the big guns. American food manufacturers' groups began frantic lobbying in Washington. The Sugar Association threatened to "exercise every avenue available to expose the dubious nature" of the report. Its lobbying resulted in a scathing 2004 letter to WHO from William Steiger, special assistant at the Department of Health and Human Services (and godson to George H. W. Bush), rejecting years of research and denying any evidence of a link between junk food and obesity. Steiger's letter questioned the scientific basis for "the linking of fruit and vegetable consumption to decreased risk of obesity and diabetes." He added: "There is an unsubstantiated focus on 'good' and 'bad' foods and a conclusion that specific foods are linked to non-communicable diseases and obesity . . . the assertion that heavy marketing of energy-dense foods or fast-food outlets increases the risk of obesity is supported by almost no data." Next, Secretary of Health and Human Services Tommy Thompson threatened to withhold the $406 million annual U.S. contribution to WHO unless TRS 916 was repealed. Suffice it to say, TRS 916 was deep-sixed, there is still no DRI for sugar, no sugar limit, and the world just keeps getting fatter and sicker.

Anything but a SNAP: The USDA versus Mayor Bloomberg

The disparities in metabolic syndrome between the rich and poor continue to vex government at the federal and local level because they are the ones who ultimately have to pay for it. Mayor Michael Bloomberg of New York City has been a public health pioneer and out front on this issue from the outset. In 2011, Bloomberg petitioned the SNAP program, sponsored by the USDA, to conduct a pilot project in New York City to remove sugared beverages from its portfolio. He argued that SNAP would save $4 billion a year and that the government would save countless sums on Medicaid and Medicare. Unfortunately, the USDA denied Bloomberg's petition, saying there were no outcome measures, no determination of what defined a sugared beverage, and no preparation on the part of vendors.

The USDA was also concerned that SNAP recipients would be "stigmatized."[10] Stigmatized? If you're poor and using food stamps, you're already stigmatized. If you're obese, you're already stigmatized. How much more stigmatization could the USDA argue? The goal of the SNAP program is "to provide improved levels of nutrition among low-income households." In fact, the American Beverage Association had lobbied the USDA, accusing New York City of unfair discrimination to prevent food stamps from being used to purchase sugary beverages.

The Legislative Branch: Protecting the Food Industry

The National School Lunch Program (NSLP)

More than thirty million children eat their lunch at school due to the NSLP, an entitlement of the Farm Bill. Children who use this program have an increased prevalence of obesity, even after race and poverty are factored in.[11] The School Meals Initiative of 1995 provides that school lunches must contain no more than 30 percent of calories from fat and 25 percent of the daily allowance of protein, calcium, iron, vitamin A, vitamin C, and age-appropriate calories. Not one word about sugar (or vitamin D, for that matter). And there's the rub. In 2010, schools were required to limit the levels of saturated fat, sodium, calories, and trans fats in meals. Still not one word about sugar. And while "whole grains" are required, they are not defined (see chapter 12).

Everyone is a dietitian, even politicians. In 1983, President Reagan determined that ketchup was a vegetable. More recently, in response to the "restrictive" guidelines placed on school lunches, lobbyists representing pizza manufacturers and cheese producers went to work. They obtained congressional concessions that one eighth of a cup of tomato paste would have the nutritional equivalent of one eighth of a cup of vegetables. In November 2011, Congress unapologetically got into the nutrition business, declaring "pizza is now a vegetable." Who knew?

The "Cheeseburger Bill"

In 2000, lawsuits lobbed against McDonald's for causing obesity and heart disease struck fear in the heart of Big Food. Its response was to lobby Congress to draft the Personal Responsibility in Food Consumption Act, aka the "Cheeseburger Bill." Representative Jim Sensenbrenner (R-Wisc.) exclaimed, "This bill says, 'Don't run off and file a lawsuit if you are fat.' It says, 'Look in the mirror because you're the one to blame. . . If a person knows or should know that eating copious orders of super-sized McDonald's products is unhealthy and could result in weight gain, it is not the place of the law to protect them from their own excesses.'" The bill has yet to get to the Oval Office, but it has been passed by the House of Representatives. Instead, individual states are bowing to the pressure, or the dollars. Minnesota state representative Dean Urdahl (R-Grove City) said, "It's about personal responsibility; it's about jobs; it's about protecting our food industry. It's also about helping our consumers not have to pay increased costs because of liability." Despite its passage in the state legislature, on May 27, 2011, a similar bill in Minnesota was vetoed by Governor Mark Dayton. Other states are maneuvering to pass their own versions.

Gag on This: Eat It and Shut Up

More insidiously, Representative Scott DesJarlais (R-Tenn.), a physician himself, in 2012 introduced H.R. 3848, the "Protecting Foods and Beverages from Government Attack Act of 2012," which would prohibit the use of federal money for advertising campaigns against anything on the FDA's GRAS list. Agriculture gag rules have been around for decades; this is how Oprah got into trouble for disparaging meat. But Representative DesJarlais' bill completely misses the point. As an example, if he has his way and succeeds in making you say no to trans fats—despite all the science, it's still on the GRAS list—New York City mayor Michael Bloomberg might find himself hauled into jail.

Whose Side Is Government On?

Our representatives couldn't be more duplicitous when it comes to obesity and our metabolic health. The executive and legislative branches are elected to generate dollars. Public health spends dollars. And the black hole of obesity sucks in even more dollars. Worse yet, not one diet and exercise intervention has been shown to save dollars for government. The government may as well promote policies that will make the food industry (and often themselves) more money. And that's why it continues its mantra of "personal responsibility." No wonder our citizens don't trust our government to get us out of this mess. Except that public health efforts can't and won't occur without some sort of effective societal intervention.

The Judicial Branch: No Horse in This Race

But hope is not completely lost. There's one branch of government that has not yet been co-opted: the judicial branch. The assumption is that the law is impartial—although the legislators who make new laws might not be, witness the Cheeseburger Bill—and that careful use of the law might extricate us from our current vicious cycle.[12] In 2009, at a major international public

health forum in India, the participants composed the Hyderabad Statement, which includes the sentence "All significant public health interventions involve and require the use of law."

When other public health debacles have reached a "tipping point," the
law has helped pave the way for reform by enforcing such community-
protecting features as sanitation, building standards, and pollution control.[13] Whether it's reducing greenhouse gases or testing for HIV, the law
has played a pivotal role in advancing the public health agenda. For instance, the assault against smoking began with the lawsuit brought by the
Mississippi attorney general to recoup claims. Law is blind, but could the
law help us see our way out of this mess?

Prosecution for Deceptive Advertising

The Federal Trade Commission (FTC) is charged with regulating "unfair or
deceptive" business practices, including food advertising. "Unfair" practices are those that may cause substantial, unavoidable injury (to consumers) that is not outweighed by offsetting consumer or competitive benefits.
Advertising is "deceptive" if it is likely to mislead consumers into making
decisions regarding a product. In 1972 the FTC exercised this charge effectively by prosecuting Sugar Information, a public relations arm of the
Sugar Association, with unfair advertising practices, based on the type of
ad seen here (figure 21.1), one of several that ran in newspapers nationwide. This ad suggests that you will eat fewer calories at a meal if you consume sugar before the meal, a claim whose veracity had not been examined,
and that could be detrimental if followed. Sadly, the food industry continues to find itself on the receiving end of "cease and desist" motions—
everything from a 1992 disputation that a Kraft Singles cheese slice
contained calcium equal to 5 ounces of milk to charges that advertising
claims touting a breakfast of Frosted Mini-Wheats was "clinically shown to
improve kids' attentiveness by nearly 20 percent" and removing the "boosts
immunity" claim from Kellogg's Cocoa Krispies in 2009.

Unfortunately, the FTC was declawed in 1978 when it attempted to
regulate junk food advertising in the now-infamous KidVid scandal.
Within the context of free speech, the food industry vigorously lobbied

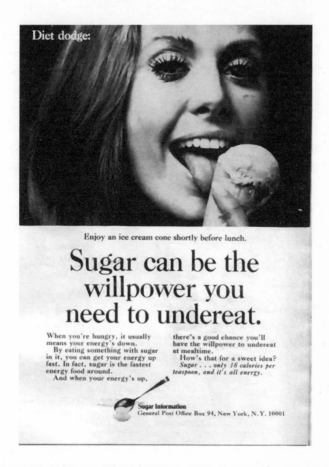

Fig. 21.1. Don't Believe Everything You Lick. A newspaper advertisement composed by Sugar Information, Inc., which was struck down by the Federal Trade Commission in 1972 for unfair advertising practices. Sugar Information, Inc., was the public information/education arm of the U.S. Sugar Association.

Congress to prevent any regulation of marketing to children, upon which Congress threatened to defund the FTC unless the matter were dropped. On the subject of regulating the food industry, the FTC has never been heard from again. The following is an excerpt from the FTC's own record: "Based on the history of FTC regulation of children's advertising . . . and the current state of the law with regard to commercial speech and the First Amendment, one can only conclude that restricting untruthful advertising is not the way to address the health concerns regarding obesity."[14]

Other Ways the Law Can Fight Obesity

The law is a powerful tool because it demands facts—something that science can supply. By nature, I'm not a litigious person, but lawsuits are a great way to get the food industry and government's attention, and maybe even to get them to do the "right thing," because the Court effectively muzzles the opposing lobbyists. Most legal action in the field of public health has revolved around the question of "negligence" or "failure to warn." Can either the food industry or institutions that push problem food onto vulnerable populations be held liable?

Various avenues for state-by-state change are being considered. For instance, lawsuits in Washington State have been successful against school boards that accept money from soft drink companies in exchange for exclusive vending rights. Other possible lawsuits with public value include going against public education officials who cut physical education from the school curriculum and against insurance health plans for not covering medically necessary weight-loss treatments. What follows are some more ideas that might have "legs" in the public health arena to help curb obesity:

Food Labeling

What about suing the FDA to revise the Nutrition Labeling and Education Act of 1990? Although food labeling has minimal effect on purchases, it couldn't hurt. The current labeling scheme, around since 1990, hasn't done anything to curb the obesity epidemic. The currents labels do not convey the important facts that the public needs to make a conscious health decision. Because what's in the food isn't important—all real foods have inherent value. What the label should tell you is what's been *added to* or *subtracted from* the food to make it more or less obesogenic. An example of such a food label scheme is presented in figure 21.2.

Alternatively, the "traffic light" food-labeling scheme is a method for influencing the nutritional quality of processed food through a simplification of the nutritional attributes of a product. Red is for products that should be consumed in small amounts or not at all (the Coca-Cola label is already red, so that should be easy), yellow for food types that should be

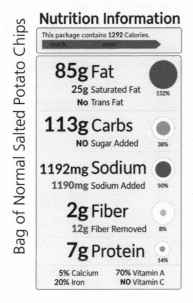
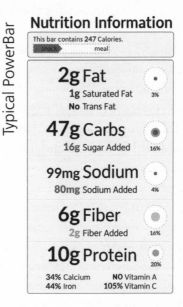

Fig. 21.2. The Lord Giveth, and Man Taketh Away. In addition to listing total nutrients, an alternative food label might include added and subtracted nutrients, to tell the whole story. Here is a sample label (courtsey of Joey Brunelle, Goose Rock Design):

a) Total calories are listed in plain language. No more "servings"—real units used instead (e.g., "this package" or "this bar").

b) Calories represented visually in a scale of a recommended snack or meal.

c) Major nutritional components listed in readable text.

d) "Sugar added," "sodium added," "fiber removed," and "fiber added" suggest the degree of processing.

e) Recommended daily values are represented visually by filled circles: the colored circle's area is proportional to the daily value (the dashed circle).

f) The circles could be colored according to their dietary desirability. Added sugar, added salt, and omega-6 and trans fats could be in red. Natural sugar and natural sodium could be in yellow. Fiber could be in green.

g) If there is none of an item, it is listed in plain language, as in "No Trans Fat" or "No Vitamin A."

h) Color and size of the circle signal how healthy a particular food item is.

consumed in moderation (for instance, whole grains), and green for food that can be consumed anytime (vegetables, fruits). This method could be applied to three nutritional areas of common concern to the public at large: fat, sugar, and salt. The more green lights displayed, the healthier the product. The problem here is that the food industry may attempt to alter the food specifically by quantitative tinkering with its nutrient profile.

Take Dietary Control Away from the USDA

MyPlate, which replaced the USDA's Food Pyramid, calls for 50 percent fruits and vegetables, 25 percent whole grain carbohydrate, and 25 percent protein. A marked improvement and, as an aside, almost identical to the "plate model" our clinic at UCSF has used for the last nine years. But the USDA still forges nutrition policy, which is still faulty.

In 2008, I stood for membership on the 2010 Dietary Guidelines Advisory Committee (DGAC). I asked my friend and 2005 DGAC chairperson, Janet King, if she was going to stand for membership again and she said, "Absolutely not. I'm tired and frustrated." She elaborated: "Our Committee submitted a 480-page document. Of those, there were 80 pages on sugar and 80 pages on fiber. When the final document was approved by the USDA, the document was 80 pages total, and the sections on both sugar and fiber were gone." "How can they do that? Didn't you have any recourse?" I asked. "We're an advisory committee," she said. "We have no teeth."

The question is, why is the USDA in charge of the country's nutrition anyway? In 2003 the *Chicago Tribune* reported the comments of Senator Peter Fitzgerald (R-Ill.)[15]: "The primary mission of the USDA is, after all, to promote the sale of agricultural products . . . So putting the USDA in charge of dietary advice is in some respects like putting the fox in charge of the henhouse." So who should be in charge of our nutrition? How about *anyone* without a vested interest in pushing the poison?

Sue the FDA to Remove Fructose from the GRAS List

Ultimately, food producers and distributors must reduce the amount of sugar added to foods. But sugar is cheap, tastes good, and sells, so companies have little incentive to change. The FDA could "set the table" for change by removing fructose from the GRAS list. Opponents will argue that other nutrients on the GRAS list, such as iron and vitamins A and D, can also be toxic when overconsumed. However, unlike sugar, these substances have no abuse potential. Sugar's removal from the GRAS list would send a powerful signal to the European Food Safety Authority and the rest of the world, and would force the food industry to rethink its recipes.

While, according to FDA regulations, the GRAS status of a substance must be reconsidered as new scientific information emerges, the agency has not systematically reconsidered GRAS substances since the 1980s.[16] For instance, despite overwhelming evidence, the FDA has largely not responded to concerns about trans fats, despite eleven citizen petitions submitted to the agency between 2004 and 2008. There is more than enough evidence to bring sugar to a new review by the FDA. Can the FDA rethink sugar as not GRAS? It can, but it won't without a lot of pressure—the kind that comes from a lawsuit. Its own rules keep it from acting. The following comes from the tobacco industry documents, written by an executive for Philip Morris, about the limits in challenging the poisonous nature of food:

> A food shall be deemed to be adulterated if it bears or contains any poisonous or deleterious substance which may render it injurious to health . . . [such that] food products does not result in acute injuries such as poisoning, and with preventing consumers from being misled, *but not with the prevention of chronic diseases even though its own regulations explicitly postulate the connection between such products and such diseases.* (italics mine)

In other words, the FDA is concerned only with *acute* toxins in food (those chemicals that kill you immediately), not *chronic* toxins, which kill you slowly by promoting chronic disease. Fructose is a chronic dose-dependent toxin, so, unless the FDA is forced, don't expect it to initiate any changes on its own. Petitions don't work. Lawsuits do.

Trusting Government, and Ourselves

None of the suggestions in this chapter is remotely actionable today, because government has been co-opted in what is known as "elite capture." By this we mean that the government bends the regulatory systems in the food industry's favor, to maintain a decidedly lopsided power structure. Either the legislative branch won't act because the food industry is paying it off, the executive branch won't act because it's afraid of the political repercussions, or the populace won't act because as far as they are concerned, "a calorie is still a calorie" and they still believe in personal responsibility—and they're addicted anyway. Our current distrust of government is well placed. It's in our DNA. Thomas Jefferson said, "That government is best which governs the least, because its people discipline themselves." Yet there is no discipline. That's the curse of addiction.

So we're now faced with a highly unpleasant lesser of two evils. The question is not whether you have any control over your food. You don't. The question is, who do you want to abdicate to? Whom do you want in your kitchen? The government, which will co-opt your rights and your wallet, or the food industry, which has already co-opted your rights, your wallet, and your health? I guess we all have to get really sick first and have no other options. The bottom has to fall out. And then it's time for societal rehab. We're just about there.

Chapter 22

A Call for Global Sugar Reduction

———————•———————

"This unprecedented meeting—the first ministerial conference on non-communicable diseases—is evidence of a new and positive trend: the world is paying attention to non-communicable diseases as never before . . . Chronic illnesses influenced by diet, tobacco consumption and other individual behaviors were long thought to be diseases of affluence. That is clearly not the case. The World Health Organization estimates that nearly 9 out of 10 people who die from non-communicable diseases under the age of 60 live in the developing world. They have less protection from the risks and consequences of these diseases than people in the developed world."

—U.N. secretary-general Ban-Ki Moon, to the First
Global Ministerial Conference on Healthy Lifestyles and
Noncommunicable Disease Control, Moscow, April 28, 2011

It Tolls for Thee . . .

On September 20, 2011, in New York, the UN secretary-general lowered the boom. The world is dying. Not of the plague, not of influenza, not of Ebola, not of AIDS. Noncommunicable disease (i.e., heart disease, diabetes, cancer, dementia—in other words, the metabolic syndrome) is now a greater threat to the developed *and* developing world than is infectious disease. This is quite a paradigm shift. The reality is that every country that has adopted the Western diet (now the industrial global diet) has witnessed rising rates of obesity and metabolic syndrome. Furthermore, economic development means that the populations of low- and middle-income countries are living longer (which is a good thing), but are therefore more susceptible to these diseases (which is a bad thing). Currently, there are 30 percent more obese than undernourished people on the planet. And 80 percent of deaths from heart disease and other noncommunicable diseases occur in low- and middle-income countries.[1]

The Rationale for Targeting Sugar

The UN announcement targets tobacco, alcohol, and diet as the central risk factors in noncommunicable disease. The first two, tobacco and alcohol, by everyone's estimation, are the most prevalent and dangerous chronic exposures on the planet. Both are regulated by governments around the world to protect the public health—not just for the abuser, but for the innocent bystander as well. Alcohol has a long history of governmental control, extending back to ancient China, when an attempt was made to curb alcohol's promotion of unruly behavior and property damage. More recently, the efforts of MADD (Mothers Against Drunk Driving) and other advocacy groups have promoted efforts to curtail drunk driving, more to protect the innocent bystander than the drinker himself. Public outcry works. Tobacco is more recently regulated, not just because of lung cancer, but also to curtail the dangers of secondhand smoke. But what, if anything, about diet should be targeted? And why? This is a little more complicated. Unlike with tobacco and alcohol, we *need* food. What aspect of the Western diet should be targeted for intervention?

Denmark took the first plunge, despite the fact that obesity isn't a huge problem there. The Danes first chose to tax foods high in saturated fat, even though most medical professionals no longer believe that fat is the primary culprit (see chapter 10). After all, look where such a belief has gotten us. But now Denmark is ready to tax sugar as well, which, as you will see, is a much more plausible and defensible step.

Do we really need to restrict sugar? After all, sugar is fun. Sugar is family. Sugar is pleasure. Coke's 2009 tag line is "Open Happiness." Now, that's going a bit too far. Maybe pleasure, on a good day. But there's nothing "happy" about sugar, and this book documents the unhappiness that sugar has wrought worldwide.

In 2003 a landmark book called *Alcohol: No Ordinary Commodity*[2] laid out the four criteria that the public health community established to justify the regulation of a substance: unavoidability, toxicity, abuse, and costs to society. Alcohol and tobacco easily meet these criteria. But what about sugar? My colleagues Laura Schmidt, Claire Brindis, and I evaluated these effects.[3]

Unavoidability

Sugar is now the most ubiquitous foodstuff worldwide, and has been added to virtually every processed food, limiting consumer choice and the ability to avoid it. Approximately 80 percent of the 600,000 consumer packaged foods in the United States have added caloric sweeteners. The only way you can avoid it is if you grow your own. Many schools have removed soda from their vending machines but they still serve juice and chocolate milk. When you were five, would you opt for water over chocolate milk? And in 40 percent of schools in California there are no drinking water fountains, so again, your children don't get to choose, and can't avoid the sugar.[4] Daily sugar intake in many countries now tops 400 calories (see chapter 11).

Toxicity

If "a calorie is a calorie" were true, and obesity and metabolic syndrome were a result of "empty calories," the mantra of "eat less, exercise more" would stand. But sugar is not "empty calories." The fructose component is a toxin by itself—a chronic one, a dose-dependent one—but a toxin nonetheless.[5] We know about the ill effects of smoking and prolonged alcohol usage. Every single disease or condition of metabolic syndrome is driven by fructose, including hypertension, through increases in uric acid; high triglycerides and insulin resistance, through synthesis of fat in the liver; diabetes, via increased liver glucose production combined with insulin resistance; accelerated aging, due to damage to lipids and protein; likely cancer, due to DNA damage, high insulin levels, and the fact that some cancers seem to use fructose preferentially for energy; and likely dementia, through insulin resistance in the brain.

Abuse

Sugar acts on the reward center[6] to encourage subsequent intake (see chapters 5 and 11). Whether it fits the criterion for addiction is irrelevant; the stuff is abused. You get hooked at an early age, and it's harder to kick the habit after years of prolonged usage. There are now numerous human studies examining the dependence-producing properties of sugar.[7] By reducing dopamine signaling in the brain's reward center, the pleasure derived from food is reduced (increasing tolerance), compelling the individual to consume more. And when the sugar is stopped, symptoms of irritability (withdrawal) become apparent.

Costs to Society

Society acknowledges that alcohol abuse (driving under the influence) and smoking (effects of secondhand smoke) can injure the innocent bystander. But how does your sugar consumption affect me? An extra $274 million in jet fuel to cart the obese around the skies? Discomfort on the subway? Sinking of boats due to the weight? In 2003 the *Ethan Allen*, a tour boat, capsized in Lake George, New York, because it was certified to carry 48 people at 140 pounds, yet the average person aboard was 25 percent over that weight. The diseases of metabolic syndrome are bankrupting the medical care systems of our country and the world at large.[8] In the United States, we're talking $150 billion annually in health care expenditures and $73 billion in lost productivity due to obesity in full-time employees.[9] This amount is expected to increase to $192 billion by 2030. And because 27 percent of military applicants are now rejected for obesity-related reasons, the past three U.S. surgeons general and the chairman of the U.S. Joint Chiefs of Staff have declared obesity a "threat to national security."

Why Alcohol Is So Relevant

The appropriate analogy to draw for sugar is with alcohol (see chapter 11). Let's recap.

1. Alcohol is derived from the fermentation of sugar.
2. Both are metabolized by the liver, bypassing insulin regulation to overload the mitochondria and cause metabolic abnormalities.
3. Both act as an energy source, but with a clear health cost.
4. Both are legal substances that produce harm when overused.
5. Both cause the diseases of metabolic syndrome.
6. Both are addictive, acting at the reward center of the brain, with bingeing, craving, tolerance, and withdrawal.
7. Both bring with it a stigma from overuse.
8. Both are abused by the lowest socioeconomic strata, almost certainly to stimulate pleasure, and the overwhelming burden of harm falls on them.
9. Both are treated as market commodities.
10. Both have generated powerful industry lobbies and vested interests, and have co-opted the objectivity of many government officials.

Unfortunately, moderating your sugar intake is nearly impossible given our current sugar glut. Sugar is in nearly everything you eat or drink, and you're hooked on it from childhood. Given all the metabolic, hedonic, and societal similarities to alcohol, doesn't it make sense to use the lessons learned from alcohol control policies and apply them as a template for societal approaches to sugar reduction?

Does Education Change "Behavior" for Addictive Substances?

There's no question that public health campaigns can help change attitudes, which can help change disease risk. For instance, education increased condom use to reduce HIV rates. But for alcohol, tobacco, and street drugs, most of the popular approaches to public health education don't work to curtail abuse for two reasons: because they do not do anything to reduce availability of the substance in question, and because those substances are addictive. For instance, school-based education programs have little effect on reducing alcohol consumption.[10] School-based obesity education programs to date also show limited success,[11] in part because our kids' food preferences are formed before they ever get to school and because their home environment remains constant. Teaching the child won't fix her environment. *Necessary, but not sufficient.* Ask the kid who returns from fat camp and gains all his weight back within three months.

What about public service announcements (PSAs) or counter-advertising? The recent anti-tobacco ads with amputees and tracheostomy patients are pretty stark, but they don't change tobacco availability. Thus far, alcohol PSAs have demonstrated only modest effects with respect to total alcohol consumption.[12] Despite numerous ad campaigns to combat obesity, such as those in New York City,[13] there are no data that show that PSAs *alone* are effective in reducing sugar consumption. *Necessary, but not sufficient.*

How about the latest hot idea, menu labeling? New York City was the first to require in-store labeling for consumer education. The results show that, for adults, average calorie consumption did not change with the advent of labeling changes alone—828 versus 846 calories—only 15 percent of adults altered their choices based on caloric knowledge.[14] One study compared a New York City sample population exposed to labeling with a Newark, New Jersey, sample population exposed to no labeling.[15] Guess what? No difference! Worse yet, none of the current menu-labeling initiatives even measure sugar—it's just total calories, fat, and salt. *Necessary, but not sufficient.*

This goes for food labeling as well. Remember "Smart Choices," the green checkmark that the food industry placed on products to indicate compliance with USDA food standards? Cocoa Krispies and Froot Loops bore the Smart Choice insignia. Froot Loops qualified because it met standards for fiber and vitamins A and C; and because it did not exceed limits on fat, sodium, and sugar (only 12 grams per serving—or *41 percent of the product,* that's all). The program was scrapped in 2009 due to the outcry of citizens incredulous that Froot Loops was on the list. The Environmental Working Group in 2011 published Sugar in Children's Cereals,[16] which documented the sugar content of eighty-four breakfast cereals (and while they were at it, the lack of fiber). Table 22.1 shows the worst. Incredibly, Froot Loops is only number ten! Perhaps the biggest travesty is that this information is not squarely placed on the label for all to see.

Table 22.1: The Ten Worst Children's Breakfast Cereals (from among 275)

1. Kellogg's Honey Smacks: 55.6 percent sugar by weight Ingredients: Sugar, wheat, dextrose, honey, contains 2 percent or less of vegetable oil (hydrogenated or partially hydrogenated soybean), salt, caramel color, soy lecithin, BHT for freshness.
2. Post Golden Crisp: 51.9 percent sugar
3. Kellogg's Froot Loops Marshmallow: 48.3 percent sugar
4. Quaker Oats Cap'n Crunch's OOPS! All Berries: 46.9 percent sugar
5. Quaker Oats Cap'n Crunch Original: 44.4 percent sugar
6. Quaker Oats Oh!s: 44.4 percent sugar
7. Kellogg's Smorz: 43.3 percent sugar
8. Kellogg's Apple Jacks: 42.9 percent sugar
9. Quaker Oats Cap'n Crunch's Crunch Berries: 42.3 percent sugar
10. Kellogg's Froot Loops Original: 41.4 percent sugar

Then there are government guidelines. The 2010 Dietary Guidelines Advisory Committee suggested an upper limit of 25 percent of daily calories allotted to added sugar (remember, Nutrition Facts gives you only total sugar, not added sugar). However, a recent adult study showed that when 25 percent of calories were due to added sugar, people developed worsened LDL, triglycerides, and insulin resistance within two weeks.[17]

Bottom line, although lots of effort and money have been thrown at various methods of obesity prevention at the individual education level, the results are downright disappointing.[18] When it comes right down to it, you can't change behavior with information alone, especially when you're talking about addictive substances. *Necessary, but not sufficient.* Because the biochemical drive will eventually overcome any cognitive attempt to control it. Nope, it's going to be all about changing the environment, and that means changing availability.

Changing Marketing to Children: Not Much Better

There is plenty of evidence that the cumulative effect of alcohol advertising alters young people's perceptions, and encourages pro-alcohol attitudes and greater consumption.[19] While population studies find some small effects for alcohol advertising bans, individual studies of short-term impacts on alcohol consumption find no effect.[20] Worse yet, industry-sponsored efforts are even less efficacious for the public health—"Don't drink and drive," by Budweiser, has become "Drink Budweiser and then let someone else drive." Government-imposed regulations on the marketing and promotion of alcohol products have mainly targeted youth, with varied results.

Although commercials for alcohol (except for beer and wine) have been scaled back since the 1970s, messages about alcohol still pervade the airwaves. Government-imposed regulations on marketing of alcohol to youth have been somewhat effective. The success of regulations that limit how alcohol is advertised and marketed has immediate relevance for sugar reduction.

Can we limit junk food advertising, especially those marketing sugar? Marketing to children is a major goal of the food industry, as it hastens "branding" of specific products, which the child will likely take into adulthood. All this despite the fact that children can't tell the TV show from the commercial until they are eight years old. A 2007 study showed that the average American child sees thirty thousand TV commercials annually marketing fast food or candy.[21] An average of one food commercial is shown every five minutes during Saturday morning cartoons. Advertisers spent more than $10 billion targeting children and youth though TV ads, coupons, contests, public relations promotions, and packaging designed for children. All this advertising translates into purchasing requests[22] and, more important to the industry, increased consumption.[23]

In 2007 the health ministers of fifty-two European nations convened in Istanbul and agreed to ban the marketing of junk food to children.[24] Heartened by this effort, in October 2007, I asked Deborah Taylor Tate, then commissioner of the Federal Communications Commission under President George W. Bush, whether this was feasible in America. Her response was "I expect the food industry to police itself." When left to their own devices, cigarette ads blatantly targeted children until public outcry demanded that the government step in. Metabolic syndrome is currently claiming more lives than lung cancer. Clearly public outcry has to become so deafening that the government has no recourse but to take action. Against all odds, and led by Dr. Guido Gerardi Lavin, a pediatrician and former president of the Senate, the nation of Chile in May 2012 became the first nation to ban junk food marketing to children.

In 2007 the Better Business Bureau produced a voluntary industry agreement called the Children's Food and Beverage Advertising Initiative (CFBAI), which ostensibly limits advertising and promotion to children in schools, and is set to go into effect in 2014. The standards would apply equally to all companies that participate (currently seventeen), but participation is voluntary. For instance, Nestlé, the world largest food conglomerate, has thus far said, "Go fly." Here's an example of what's okay to market under this initiative: Pepperidge Farm Goldfish, Kellogg's Apple Jacks, and ConAgra's Chef Boy-ar-dee canned pastas. Not entirely happy with this response, in 2011 Congress directed the FTC, the FDA, the CDC, and the USDA to establish an Interagency Working Group (IWG) of federal nutrition, health, and marketing experts. The IWG came up with stricter, but still voluntary, guidelines that would limit not only television but also other forms of multimedia advertising (e.g., websites, online games, social media movies). The food industry lobbied Congress so hard that the IWG has withdrawn, and is planning to support the weaker, self-anointed CFBAI. So will Toucan Sam and Tony the Tiger bite the dust? Don't bet on it.[25]

Thus far, there are no government-imposed bans on the marketing of high-sugar-content products to children in the United States. Even so, despite vigorous lobbying by the food industry, San Francisco recently instituted a ban on including toys with fast food meals. Why does a toddler need more coercion to eat fast food than the food itself? Since then, the political fallout has resulted in three states banning "toy bans." Nonetheless, in June 2012 Disney got the memo—they will cease marketing of junk food to children under twelve. Hope springs eternal.

Changing the Environment

What will it really take to reduce sugar consumption? We can't get rid of it; rather, like alcohol and tobacco, we will have to learn to "peacefully co-exist" with these substances. Let's look to the many generations of international experience with alcohol control to find models that do work. Anything that works does so by limiting availability.[26] This means upstream strategies that limit supply, rather than downstream approaches that hope to decrease demand, but can't. Reducing availability can be done at three levels: taxation, restriction, and interdiction. Well, forget interdiction—that's a non-starter. It didn't work for alcohol. Criminalizing a substance as widespread or as popular as sugar would be equally doomed to failure; can you imagine sugar prohibition, with candy speak-easys and bathtubs of Coca-Cola? But successful interventions all share a common end point: curbing availability. In other words, control the environment, not behavior.

Some municipalities have taken up the gauntlet. For instance, in California we have State Bill 19, or "Sodas out of Schools." In 2008, former president Bill Clinton and former Arkansas governor Mike Huckabee reached an agreement with the beverage industry to get sodas out of schools—but they didn't negotiate the elimination of the juice and the sports drinks. In 2012 a study showed that in the twelve states where soda had been removed from schools, sugared beverage consumption by teens remained just as high as it had ever been.[27]

Taxation

Taxation is a simple and effective, if unpopular, way of reducing consumption of virtually anything. Taxation follows the law of supply and demand: adding a tax increases the price of the substance of concern such that consumers can afford to buy less of it. Alcohol taxes are popular worldwide because they are relatively cheap and easy to collect, while causing little market distortion. Alcohol taxation, in the form of special excise duties (taxing the producer), or value added and sales taxes (taxing the consumer), has proven among the most prodigious and effective ways worldwide to reduce the overall volume of drinking and, in turn, alcohol-attributable harm.[28]

Could taxing sugar help solve obesity?[29] This is one of the most incendiary topics on the agenda. Want to stop a dialogue in the United States? Utter the phrase "soda tax." Soda is not all sugar-sweetened beverages (SSBs)—SSBs are only 33 percent of all added sugar—and SSBs are not the sole cause of the obesity epidemic, so this strategy is incomplete at best.[30] Nonetheless, SSBs have several characteristics that make them the most promising target for prevention of obesity and metabolic syndrome[31] (see chapter 9). First, SSBs are a clearly defined category, unlike other "junk foods" that might contain some protein, fiber, or micronutrients. There is *nothing* in an SSB that's valuable. Oh, some will argue that juice has vitamin C. But the fiber was the good part of the fruit, and vitamin C deficiency (scurvy) is now so rare that cases of it are reported in medical journals.[32] Second, SSBs contribute more calories to the diet than any other single type of food or beverage. Third, the evidence supporting an association between SSB intake and obesity is stronger than for any other single foodstuff.

State-sponsored soft drink excise taxes reduced soft drink sales and consumption among children and adolescents, while consumption of whole milk increased. (One downside is that consumption of fruit juice also increased.)[33] Another intervention in a hospital cafeteria showed that increasing the price of a soda by 35 percent resulted in a 26 percent reduction in consumption.[34] Thus, soda taxation represents a viable public health strategy.[35] Already, Canada imposes a GST (goods and services tax), and some European countries impose a VAT (value added tax) on some sweetened foods.

In the United States, the concept of a soda tax has met with a firestorm of antagonism, from everyone from the libertarians claiming consumer freedom, to the ACLU claiming discrimination based on poverty, to the food industry claiming "scientific McCarthyism." The beverage industry has spent millions of dollars on lobbying against an SSB "sin tax." It is so desperate to derail this legislation that it offered the city of Philadelphia $10 million, including an obesity professorship at Children's Hospital of Philadelphia, if the city agreed to abandon its proposed excise tax on soda. While this offer might seem generous, Philadelphia would have raised $77 million in revenues in one year, with $20 million going toward obesity prevention, if the tax had gone through. Money talks, science walks.

A Bad Rap?

Soda taxation has gotten a bad rap for three major reasons. First, how can the poor finance a soda tax? "Regressive" taxes place a greater burden of cost on lower-income consumers.[36] The U.S. has a strong tradition of consumer rights protection; taxes that exert unfair constraints on individual choice are bad enough, and those levied on the poor are doomed to fail. Which begs the question—can a "regressive" tax be in the public health interest? Hey, it works for tobacco and alcohol. Of course it can, but with three caveats. First, regressive taxes makes sense only if the substance being taxed causes disproportionate health harms in the poor. This is certainly true for all addictive substances, including tobacco, alcohol and sugar. Remember, fructose is not an essential nutrient, the burden of metabolic syndrome is highest in lower-income minorities,[37] and the current loss of productivity and added medical costs associated with metabolic syndrome provide a strong case for widespread taxpayer benefits.

Second, the proceeds of the tax must be diverted back to the public health of the lower-income population, to balance out the regressive nature of the tax. In the case of sugar, tax revenues could be applied toward subsidies on fresh produce. They could also be used to finance commercial loan and development programs encouraging grocery stores and farmers' markets to relocate to underserved low-income communities or food deserts. By redirecting subsidies to make healthful products accessible to low-income consumers, valid concerns about regressive taxation and government paternalism can be headed off at the pass. Everyone wins (except the beverage industry).

Third, what is the purpose of the tax? To prevent obesity or to pay for obesity programs? The fear is that the politicians will abscond with the money as a quick fix to close their budget shortfalls and avoid cuts to critical services such as public safety and transportation. The American Beverage Association says that despite the rhetoric of elected officials wanting to curb obesity, soda taxes are all about filling up public coffers. Larry Young,

CEO of Dr. Pepper Snapple and chairman of the ABA, told Goldman Sachs, "You say it's for obesity. Come on, it's to fill a budget deficit." And there's real reason to be worried about this. The current proposal is for a penny-per-ounce soda tax, which would raise the price of a can of soda by $0.12. While this would generate approximately $13 billion in revenue,[38] it is unlikely to have a significant impact on reducing SSB consumption and the diseases associated with metabolic syndrome. Rather, statistical modeling suggests that the price would have to double to reduce soda consumption—so a one-dollar can of soda should cost two dollars.[39] And no one is ready for that ... yet. But give it time. No one in New York was ready to spend $11.90 for a pack of cigarettes either. Hefty taxes are required to reduce consumption of addictive substances.

Restriction of Access

Throughout this book, I've hammered one issue time and again: *control the environment*. Nothing reduces sugar consumption better than reducing sugar availability. And that means restricting access. Especially to children. We've been largely successful with alcohol. Why not sugar?

Successful alcohol control strategies restrict accessibility to purchase, such as reducing the hours retailers are open, controlling the location and density of retail markets, and limiting who can legally purchase alcohol.[40] A reasonable parallel for sugar would be tighten licensing requirements on vending machines and snack bars that sell sugary products in schools and workplaces. Many schools have removed soda from vending machines, but usually replace them with juice and sports drinks, which are no better.

Reduction in the number and density of convenience stores that sell alcohol clearly cuts down on consumption, especially in poor neighborhoods.[41] Similarly, states could apply zoning ordinances to control the number of fast food outlets and convenience stores in low-income communities, and especially around schools, while providing incentives for the establishment of grocery stores and farmers' markets. They could also apply zoning ordinances to inconvenience the food trucks that are multiplying like flies outside schools during lunchtime and after the bell rings, targeting our children. Another option would be to limit sales in stores during times of school operation, so kids couldn't buy a soda on the way home. One would expect that kids who walk to school would have lower BMIs because they exercise. Wrong. My colleague Kristine Madsen showed that kids who walk to school have higher BMIs because they're stopping to buy soda and chips![42]

Lastly, how about an age limit (such as seventeen) in order to purchase drinks with added sugar? Yes, card kids for Coke! You got a problem with that? Store managers already do it for alcohol, and it would cost nothing to implement. If parents want their kids to have a soda, they can buy it for them. Recently, parents in South Philadelphia took this upon themselves. They formed a posse by lining up outside convenience stores and blocking children from entering these stores after school.[43] Why couldn't a public health directive do the same?

Not one to be stymied by the USDA over the 2011 Food Stamp debacle, in June 2012 Mayor Michael Bloomberg unveiled a bold proposal to eliminate Big Gulps from New York City, a move well within his purview. Will this edict really reduce sugar consumption? What's to prevent people from buying two sodas instead of one? I recall a Bill DeOre cartoon from the *Dallas Morning News*, showing a kid at a fast food counter. Before downsizing, he orders a large order of fries. After, he orders sixteen orders of fries. Libertarians have gone ballistic decrying Bloomberg's usurping of personal freedom. Environmentalists are angry as this may mean more plastic waste. Politicians argue this will be unwieldy to administer. But if Bloomberg did nothing else, he sent a loud and clear message: public health is a noble cause, and one worth fighting for.

Curb the Subsidies? Or Curb the Deregulation?

In order to balance the U.S. budget, the Farm Bill needs to lose $23 billion from its ledger. Crop subsidies account for $6 billion per year; of that, $3.5 billion goes to corn, and $1.6 billion goes to soybeans. Diverting money away from subsidies is not without its dangers, especially now that we live in a global economy. One product of our corn subsidy is the production of ethanol as an additive for gasoline, but environmentalists have railed against this practice for years, as it puts more carbon emissions into the atmosphere.

There are two types of subsidies: payments to farmers only when the price of the crop is low (to keep them from going out of business), and payments to farmers based on performance, regardless of price. Over the five years from 2006 through 2011, the price of corn has never been higher[44] yet the corn subsidy continues unabated.

Propping up consumption of specific foodstuffs with price subsidies is a great way to cause market distortion. If supply and demand work their magic, then stopping a subsidy should raise prices, and our food should get more expensive. Is that good or bad? Advocates for the poor would lobby immediately. So would Iowa. But the government and the poor would ultimately save on the subsidy, in medical costs and improved worker productivity. One problem with removing these subsides is that they are unlikely to make a significant difference in the price of junk food. Furthermore, as the poor frequently have limited access to healthy alternatives, they will have to buy junk food even if the price goes up marginally. Taxation proponents favor an excise tax concept because it passes the cost on to industry, which can well afford it. The question is whether it would alter industry's practices.

A different line of reasoning suggests that it's not the subsidies that overproduce commodity crops, and overproduction is not the cause of obesity. Unlike with other industries, agricultural producers do not respond to price signals by reducing the amount of a crop when prices are low. [45] Producers may reduce hired labor, but not production. In an agricultural policy dating back to President Roosevelt's New Deal, the USDA paid farmers not to grow certain crops to prevent overproduction. To keep farms from going out of business, Congress recently approved an annual $20 billion payment to farmers as a direct subsidy, despite the increase in price of all commodities from 2006 through 2011. And no Midwest state will put the brakes on this gravy train. If the United States completely eliminated all commodity protection and subsidy policies, very few foods would change in price. But the one food that would be affected would be sugar, with a reduction in production of 33 percent (because of the elimination of the corn subsidy) and a reduction in price of 15 percent (because of the end of the sugar tariffs).[46] The point is that even though we pay more for sugar because of the sugar tariffs, we still consume more, because of sugar's abuse potential. Again, standard economic principles do not apply to addictive substances.

There's only one answer that the farmers, the food industry, and the populace can live with: differential subsidization. Instead of subsidizing corn and soy (commodity crops that are storable), why can't we subsidize something green? We have the technology to do this. When broccoli and carrots are cheaper than potato chips, then Michael Pollan's thesis on the price of a calorie can be turned around for everyone's benefit. Promotion of high-fiber foods in U.S. low-income programs such as WIC, SNAP, and NSLP would be the obvious place to start. Furthermore, growing green food means growing local. It would also make tariffs on imported goods a less important concern, because they wouldn't be subsidizing "commodities." They would be subsidizing real food.

Differential subsidization goes for water as well. In the developing world, inhabitants have three choices—drink the dangerous water, buy an in-home chlorination system, or buy "safe" sugared beverages made locally by Coke or Pepsi. If the water chlorination system is provided for free, usage is at 80 percent. If people have to buy it, they drink the sugared beverages instead, which costs more in the long term, both in money and in medical costs.[47] Until potable water is free, the developing world will continue to suffer at the hands of the food industry as well.

Like a Phoenix out of the Ashes . . .

Any of these interventions would of necessity require a new business model—one that supports real food over processed food. After all, we need the food industry; we just don't need their current fare. Because high-fiber foods have a limited shelf life, such interventions would have to support local food production and reduced use of antibiotics and pesticides, which would have implications for mitigating global warming and environmental pollution. These interventions would require allocating new farmland around the country that could be adapted to grow real food, with minimal technological prowess. However, this would of necessity require new delivery and distribution systems, and new pricing strategies. It would also require changes in marketing, especially to children. As distasteful as it is, such upstream societal interventions can be accomplished only with governmental support. (There's just no way around it.)

Reducing sugar consumption will not be easy—particularly in the emerging markets of developing countries, where soft drinks are cheaper than milk or potable water. Societal intervention is needed to reduce the supply and eventual demand for sugar. Despite the obvious medical, social, and economic benefits, we face an uphill political battle against a powerful sugar and food processing lobby, and against those in government who are already corrupted. Any change will require active engagement from all stakeholders. And that means you. Especially you. With enough public clamor, tectonic shifts in policy do become possible. Take, for instance, bans on smoking in public, the use of designated drivers, airbags in cars, and condom dispensers in public bathrooms. All unfathomable thirty years ago. Your voice changed the world. It can be a new world . . . yet again.

Epilogue: Not a Top-Down,
but a Bottom-Up Movement

———————•———————

"Politics is the entertainment branch of industry."

—Frank Zappa

In the preceding chapters, I have attempted to link the science of the obesity pandemic to existing policy. In the process, I hope I have provided a new thought process and a new direction, by looking backward. What is clear is that the few are profiting by playing the politics of obesity to their advantage, at the expense of the many. We've seen this movie before. We saw it with tobacco. The science was subverted for years before the tobacco documents laid bare the corruption of the industry. Not only did the industry consistently hide its findings, but as my UCSF colleagues Marcia Wertz and Stanton Glantz found, the industry's malfeasance even encompassed fabricating and doctoring data,[1] which, in the scientific world, is the greatest of crimes. Time for the trial.

How does a district attorney ascribe culpability? There are three components to successful prosecution. The first is association, the second is motive, and the slam-dunk is the smoking gun. Recall the fight with Big Tobacco. The association between smoking and lung cancer dates to 1964, with the first surgeon general's report. The motive became clear in the 1980s, when research documented the action of nicotine on the brain's addiction center. But it wasn't until a whistleblower pointed the way to the now-famous smoking gun documents that Big Tobacco's callous disregard for its own customers was exposed.

Does this analogy work for Big Food? The association of our food environment with obesity and metabolic syndrome is incontrovertible. We even have causation. Motive is also a no-brainer. The American food industry produces 3,900 calories per person per day, with about 29 percent wastage, but we should rationally eat 1,800–2,000. Who eats the difference? We do! Throughout evolution, humans could eat only a fixed amount, but today that amount is limitless. Because, as this book has shown, the high-sugar, low-fiber industrial global diet actually makes us hungrier! What about the smoking gun? Consider the extent to which Big Food *is* Big Tobacco (Philip Morris became Altria, which used to own Kraft General Foods; RJR Tobacco Company was once part of RJR Nabisco). Does the food industry know what it's doing? Does it know it has hijacked our evolutionary biochemistry, for its benefit and to our detriment? We'll probably never find the smoking gun for obesity, as the industry has learned its lesson about leaving stray documents around. But we've already lost one generation of kids. It's time to hold Big Food's feet to the fire, to compel it to undo what it has done to our diet in the name of "progress" and "profit." Given what it (and we) know now, if it doesn't change, that will be the smoking gun.

But there will be no prosecutions. Big Tobacco was convicted by a federal judge of RICO racketeering, and tobacco executives lost their jobs for lying to Congress. They were investigated for perjury, but none went to jail, nor were any forced to pay penalties. Huge civil settlements generated windfalls for state governments, but nothing for you. Still not convinced? Let's take another example, the economic collapse of 2008. The corporate CEOs were guilty as hell, but not one went to jail. The government financed $777 billion for corporate bailouts, but none for you. Likewise, there's no chance that any food company executive will ever be held liable. Hell, what they're doing is legal!

Worse yet, the executive and legislative branches of our government are clearly lined up behind the food industry. The Farm Bill subsidizes the commodity crops that are killing us, and the USDA continues to promote the U.S. food industry both here and abroad. And the judicial branch hasn't acted yet, in part because the public hasn't mobilized, as they still believe "*a calorie remains a calorie*"—for now.

No, my friends, this won't be solved from the top-down. This will have to be a bottom-up movement. You can't expect government to do the right thing. You have to coerce it into doing the right thing. When there are more votes at stake than dollars, that's when legislators will come around. But that's not a reason to be daunted. In a democracy, the public has power. A good example is seat belts. Today you'd never consider getting behind the wheel without fastening your seat belt, but this notion is relatively new. Although the U.S. federal mandate to fit cars with seat belts was passed in 1968, there was no federal mandate to use them. The first mandatory seat belt law was enacted in Australia in 1970. Did Australia know that wearing seat belts would save lives? No. It hadn't been done before. It just seemed like a good public health measure. The Big Three fought seat belt laws for years, and U.S. passengers continued to die. It wasn't until Mothers Against Drunk Driving made such a stink in every statehouse that mandatory seat belt laws started appearing from 1984 through 1993. To this day, seat belt legislation consists of fifty state mandates, with nothing at the federal level. A bottom-up movement that worked. And there are many more examples—smoking bans in public places, toxic waste cleanups, narcotics enforcement.

Public outcry is a powerful force for change. And it can work in obesity. I am proud to be part of an advocacy group in Walnut Creek, California, called the Wellness City Challenge (www.wellnesscitychallenge.com), led by chef Cindy Gershen. This woman is a true force of nature. Espousing real food to combat disease and promote happiness, she has almost single-handedly mobilized the Mayor's Office, the Chamber of Commerce, the Board of Education, Kaiser Permanente and other hospitals, the Restaurant Association, the local Safeway supermarkets, and SYSCO (the food procurement company) to completely retool every public food venue in the cities of Martinez and Concord for one year. The vending machines have been restocked with apples and oranges, and there's nary a soda to be found. As part of the intervention, students at Mount Diablo High School are learning to cook by serving real food for the teachers at breakfast. The kids can't believe the teachers are losing weight and happy to come to work and teach; and now they themselves want the real food instead of the stuff from their traditional fast food concessions. This demonstration project has many supporters, including the American Heart Association, and has caught the eye of many benefactors, who see the power in the message.

Hopefully you do, too. While this book is about the dispassionate science and logic of obesity and how it can help individuals and society, I'm a human being as well. I get sick when I think of what's happened to us, our country, and our planet. This book is my outcry for a better world for our children. Time to cry out—and just maybe our children will Inherit the Earth.

ACKNOWLEDGMENTS

While I am responsible for everything this book says, I didn't come to all its conclusions by myself. I have scores of collaborators, and people to acknowledge and thank. And they deserve to take a bow.

My journey into the world of obesity began sixteen years ago at St. Jude Children's Research Hospital in Memphis, where Tom Merchant, Melissa Hudson, Pam Hinds, Robbin and Mike Christensen, Shengjie Wu, Xiaoping Xiong, Bob Danish, Randi Schreiber, Susan Post, Susan Rose, and George Burghen were instrumental in the initial work in children with obesity due to brain tumors. At the University of Tennessee, I am indebted to Pedro Velasquez-Meyer, Kathy Spencer, Beth Connelly, Ann Cashion, Cynthia Buffington, and Judy Soberman for our initial adult observations.

The majority of the work and the formulations espoused in this book stem from my last eleven years at the University of California, San Francisco. I have stellar colleagues in the Weight Assessment for Teen and Child Health (WATCH) program, including Andrea Garber, Kristine Madsen, Patrika Tsai, Cam-Tu Tran, Luis Rodriguez, Joan Valente, Lisa Groesz, Hannah Thompson, Michael Gonzaga, Maria Martin, Diane Luce, Meghan Gould, Frank Brodie, Rachel Lipman, Kelly Jordan, and Sally Elliott. These are the people who have done the heavy lifting, and also the ones who keep me honest. My colleagues studying stress and addiction in the Center for Obesity Assessment, Study and Treatment (COAST) are Elissa Epel, Barbara Laraia, Nancy Adler, Rick Hecht, Peter Bacchetti, Nancy Hills, Janet

Tomiyama, Laurel Mellin, Naomi Stotland, and Mel Heyman. Our fructose work is a team effort between UCSF (Kathy Mulligan, Sue Noworolski, Viva Tai, and Mike Wen) and Touro University (Jean-Marc Schwarz and Alejandro Gugliucci). At University of California at Berkeley, I am indebted to members of the Center for Weight and Health (CWH), including Pat Crawford, Lorene Ritchie, Gail Woodward-Lopez, Sharon Fleming, Joanne Ikeda, George Brooks, Aarthi Raman, and Sushma Sharma. At the UC Berkeley Center for Environmental Research and Children's Health (CERCH) are Brenda Eskenazi, Kim Harley, Asa Bradman, and Nina Holland. Our surgical work includes Diana Farmer, Shinjiro Hirose, Marco Patti, Bill Aldrich, John Kral, and at the University of Rochester, Thad Boss (deceased) and Jeff Peters. I have stellar obesity colleagues in the basic sciences at UCSF as well, in particular, Holly Ingraham, Christian Vaisse, Lynda Frassetto, Allison Xu, Eric Verdin, Bob Farese, Suneil Koliwad, Kaveh Ashrafi, and Larry Tecott, who have taught me so much. Special mention also goes to Stan Glantz and Neal Benowitz at the Center for Tobacco Research. Our advocacy work includes chef Cindy Gershen, Julie Kaufmann of the American Heart Association, Andrea Bloom of ConnectWell, and Tim Luedtke of Navigator Benefit Solutions, LLC. Our policy work includes Laura Schmidt and Claire Brindis at the UCSF Philip R. Lee Institute for Health Policy Studies, Sanjay Basu at the Stanford Prevention Institute, Jennifer Pomeranz at Yale, and internationally, Ricardo Uauy, Carlos Monteiro, Juan Rivera, Simon Barquera, and Philip James.

I would also like to acknowledge several other pediatric investigators around the world for their help and camaraderie as we all try to stem the tide of the obesity epidemic. David Ludwig (*Ending the Food Fight*), Fran Kaufman (*Diabesity*), Miriam Vos (*The No-Diet Obesity Solution for Kids*), and Peter Gluckman (*Fat, Fate, and Disease*) have already jumped into the fray with books for the public. Special acknowledgments also go to Jack Yanovski, Sonia Caprio, Dennis Styne, Silva Arslanian, Mike Freemark, Jeff Schwimmer, Dick Jackson, Ram Weiss, Martin Wabitsch, Hermann Müller, Christian Roth, Felix Kreier, Franco Chiarelli, Takehiko Ohzeki, and Ze'ev Hochberg. A call-out to Kevin Boyd of Chicago, a pediatric dentist and the world's first paleodontist. Other notables include Bruce McEwen and Rudy Leibel. And also Gary Taubes for keeping me grounded.

I also want to acknowledge two non-medical people I've never met, and who figured this stuff out by themselves without any help: David Gillespie, a lawyer from Brisbane, Australia, and Nicholas Krilanovich, a retired electrical engineer in Seattle. They deserve enormous credit for sharing their messages, and going it alone.

In particular, I want to thank an unbelievably talented and enthusiastic cadre of students, post-docs, and mentees for all their hard work, grant generation, and paper production; for their good fellowship; for putting up with me; and for making me look good. Kudos to pre-docs Renee Matos, Jessica Myers, Emily King, Jason Langheier, Annie Valente, Marcia Wertz, and Paula Yoffe. My obesity post-docs have included Chaluntorn Preeyasombat, Elvira Isganaitis, Clement Cheung, Drew Bremer, Stephanie Nguyen, Carolyn Jasik, Ivy Aslan, Lisa Goldman Rosas, Anjali Jain, and Emily Perito. Junior faculty include Jyu-Lin Chen, Anisha Patel, and Janet Wojcicki, and also some not-so-junior visiting professors: Anastasia Hadjiyannakis (Canada), Young Eun Choi (Korea), Jung Sub Lim (Korea), and Xiaonan Li (China).

This book is really the brainchild of my agent, Janis Donnaud. She found me, and convinced me that my voice was unique, that this book was necessary, and that the world needed it. Agents are usually interested in the product and the money. Not Janis. She is a thinker, a visionary. This book is the product of a three-year roller-coaster ride. Janis rode it bare-knuckled along with me and saw it to the end. Thanks as well to my editor, Amy Dietz, for her passion, humor, and unique point of view. And to my publisher, Caroline Sutton, for seeing what others couldn't. I'd also like to thank Marcia and Mark Elias and Doris Levin for critiquing the first draft of this book, Bob Hunt for historical recollections, Matt Chamberlain for his computer prowess, and Glenn Randle for his graphic genius.

But most important, I must thank my various families. First, my biological family—my wife, Julie; my daughters, Miriam and Meredith; my parents, Judy and Dick; and my sister, Carole. Aside from teaching me everything I know about genetics, they have all stood by me and loved me throughout, especially during the writing of this book on top of my day job. It seems trite to say I couldn't have done it without them, but indeed they were and always are my inspiration. And I must thank my adopted family, my colleagues at UCSF Pediatric Endocrinology; the most productive academic division with the fewest people in the country. Mel Grumbach, Felix Conte, Selna Kaplan (deceased), Steve Gitelman, Steve Rosenthal, and Saleh Adi are indeed my family—a dysfunctional one, to be sure, but family nonetheless. And lastly, I give my most special thanks to the three smartest, most logical, most scientific, fairest, most caring, and most loving people in science it is my fortune to call my friends. Without any one of them, I'd have given up long ago. First, my UCSF division head, Walter Miller, a brilliant scientist and physician with a mind like a steel trap, who has led by example, has always been supportive, and has always been there to help parse the criticisms and the politics. Second, Howard Federoff, the executive dean of Georgetown University Medical Center, perhaps the most complete human being ever to walk the earth. Howard is the ultimate role model, someone to emulate on every level. Talking science with Howard is tantamount to a religious awakening. Howard has never stopped believing in me, even when I didn't believe in myself. To be considered his friend is among the most satisfying aspects of my life. Lastly, my scientific soul sister, co-director of the Childhood Obesity Institute at Children's National Medical Center, Michele Mietus-Snyder. I'm sure if you asked her, she would tell you I taught her more than she taught me, but don't believe it. If it weren't for her scientific acumen, her critical thinking, and her genuine altruistic goodness, I seriously doubt this book would ever have taken shape.

I love you all.

NOTES

Chapter 1

1   J. Kim et al., "Trends in Overweight from 1980 Through 2001 Among Preschool-Aged Children Enrolled in a Health Maintenance Organization," *Obesity* 14 (2006): 1164–71.

2   S. J. Olshansky et al., "A Potential Decline in Life Expectancy in the United States in the 21st Century," *New Engl. J. Med.* 352 (2005): 1138–45.

3   World Health Organization, Fact Sheet: Obesity and Overweight (2011), www.who.int/mediacentre/factsheets/fs311/en/.

4   UN General Assembly, "Prevention and Control of Non-Communicable Diseases," New York, 2010.

5   J. M. Chan et al., "Obesity, Fat Distribution, and Weight Gain as Risk Factors for Clinical Diabetes in Men," *Diabetes Care* 17 (1994): 961–69.

6   S. L. Gortmaker et al., "Changing the Future of Obesity: Science, Policy, and Action," *Lancet* 378 (2011): 838–47.

7   K. C. Sung et al., "Interrelationship Between Fatty Liver and Insulin Resistance in the Development of Type 2 Diabetes," *J. Clin. Endocrinol. Metab.* 96 (2011): 1093–97.

Chapter 2

1   S. L. Gortmaker et al., "Changing the Future of Obesity: Science, Policy, and Action," *Lancet* 378 (2011) 838–47.

2   R. Padwal et al., "Long-Term Pharmacotherapy for Obesity and Overweight," Cochrane Database Syst. Rev., Art. No.: CD004094. DOI: 10.1002/14651858 (2004). PMID: 15266516.

3   C. B. Newgard et al., "A Branched-Chain Amino Acid-Related Metabolic Signature That Differentiates Obese and Lean Humans and Contributes to Insulin Resistance," *Cell Metab.* 9 (2009): 311–26.

4   P. Chanmugam et al., "Did Fat Intake in the United States Really Decline Between 1989–1991 and 1994–1996?" *J. Am. Diet. Assoc.* 103 (2003): 867–72.

Chapter 3

1   D. Thompson et al., "Lifetime Health and Economic Consequences of Obesity,"
    Arch. Int. Med. 159 (1999): 2177–83.
2   J. Bhattacharya et al., "Who Pays for Obesity?" *J. Econ. Perspect.* 25 (2011):
    139–58.
3   J. B. Schwimmer et al., "Health-Related Quality of Life of Severely Obese
    Children and Adolescents," *JAMA* 289 (2003): 1813–19.
4   T. A. Wadden et al., "Treatment of Obesity by Very Low Calorie Diet, Behavior
    Therapy, and Their Combination: A Five-Year Perspective," *Int. J. Obes.* 13
    (1989): 39–46; M. W. Schwartz et al., "Regulation of Body Adiposity and the
    Problem of Obesity," *Arterioscler. Thromb. Vasc. Biol.* 17 (1997): 233–38.
5   S. Yoo et al., "Obesity in Korean Pre-Adolescent School Children: Comparison
    of Various Anthropometric Measurements Based on Bioelectrical Impedance
    Analysis," *Int. J. Obes.* 30 (2006): 1086–90.
6   N. Gupta et al., "Childhood Obesity in Developing Countries: Epidemiology,
    Determinants, and Prevention," *Endocr. Rev.* 33 (2012): 48–70.
7   A. Ramachandran et al., "Diabetes in Asia," *Lancet* 375 (2010): 408–18.
8   B. M. Popkin, "Global Nutrition Dynamics: The World Is Shifting Rapidly
    Toward a Diet Linked with Noncommunicable Diseases," *Am. J. Clin. Nutr.* 84
    (2006): 289–98.
9   Y. C. Klimentidis et al., "Canaries in the Coal Mine: A Cross-Species Analysis of
    the Plurality of Obesity Epidemics," *Proc. Biol. Sci.* 278 (2011): 1626–32.
10 W. Park et al., "The Metabolic Syndrome: Prevalence and Associated Risk Factor
    Findings in the US Population from the Third National Health and Nutrition
    Examination Survey, 1988–1994," *Arch. Intern. Med.* 163 (2003): 427–36.
11 C. Gordon et al., "Measuring Food Deserts in New York City's Low-Income
    Neighborhoods," *Health Place* 17 (2011): 696–700.
12 M. de Onis et al., "Global Prevalence and Trends of Overweight and Obesity
    Among Preschool Children," *Am. J. Clin. Nutr.* 92 (2010): 1257–64.
13 Kaiser Family Foundation, "Food for Thought: Television Food Advertising to
    Children in the United States" (2007), www.kff.org/entmedia/upload/7618.pdf.
14 J. Kim et al., "Trends in Overweight from 1980 through 2001 Among Preschool-
    Aged Children Enrolled in a Health Maintenance Organization," *Obesity* 14
    (2006): 1164–71.
15 A. R. Cashmore, "The Lucretian Swerve: The Biological Basis of Human
    Behavior and the Criminal Justice System," *Proc. Natl. Acad. Sci.* 107 (2010):
    4499–504.

Chapter 4

1   R. H. Lustig et al., "Disorders of Energy Balance," in *Pediatric Endocrinology*,
    ed. M. Sperling (New York: Elsevier, 2008), pp. 788–838.

2   J. S. Flier, "What's in a Name? In Search of Leptin's Physiologic Role," *J. Clin. Endocr. Metab.* 83 (1998): 1407–13.

3   I. S. Farooqi et al., "Effects of Recombinant Leptin Therapy in a Child with Congenital Leptin Deficiency," *N. Engl. J. Med.* 341 (1999): 913–15.

4   R. L. Leibel, "The Role of Leptin in the Control of Body Weight," *Nutr. Rev.* 60 (2002): S15–S9.

5   R. L. Leibel et al., "Changes in Energy Expenditure Resulting from Altered Body Weight," *N. Engl. J. Med.* 332 (1995): 621–28.

6   Y. Zhang et al., "Positional Cloning of the Mouse Obese Gene and Its Human Homologue," *Nature* 393 (1994): 425–32.

7   I. S. Farooqi et al., "Genetics of Obesity in Humans," *Endocr. Rev.* 27 (2006): 710–18.

8   H. Munzberg et al., "Molecular and Anatomical Determinants of Central Leptin Resistance," *Nat. Neurosci.* 8 (2005): 566–70.

9   S. B. Heymsfield et al., "Recombinant Leptin for Weight Loss in Obese and Lean Adults: A Randomized, Controlled, Dose-Escalation Trial," *JAMA* 282 (1999): 1568–75.

10 G. A. Bray et al., "Manifestations of Hypothalamic Obesity in Man: A Comprehensive Investigation of Eight Patients and a Review of the Literature," *Medicine* 54 (1975): 301–33.

11 N. Satoh et al., "Pathophysiological Significance of the Obese Gene Product, Leptin in Ventromedial Hypothalamus (VMH)-Lesioned Rats: Evidence for Loss of Its Satiety Effect in VMH-Lesioned Rats," *Endocrinology* 138 (1997): 947–54.

12 M. G. Shaikh et al., "Reductions in Basal Metabolic Rate and Physical Activity Contribute to Hypothalamic Obesity," *J. Clin. Endocr. Metab.* 93 (2008): 2588–93.

13 R. H. Lustig et al., "Octreotide Therapy of Pediatric Hypothalamic Obesity: A Double-Blind, Placebo-Controlled Trial," *J. Clin. Endocr. Metab.* 88 (2003): 2586–92.

14 P. A. Velasquez-Mieyer et al., "Suppression of Insulin Secretion Promotes Weight Loss and Alters Macronutrient Preference in a Subset of Obese Adults," *Int. J. Obesity* 27 (2003): 219–26; R. H. Lustig et al., "A Multicenter, Randomized, Double-Blind, Placebo-Controlled, Dose-Finding Trial of a Long-Acting Formulation of Octreotide in Promoting Weight Loss in Obese Adults with Insulin Hypersecretion," *Int. J. Obesity* 30 (2006): 331–41.

15 R. H. Lustig et al., "Obesity, Leptin Resistance, and the Effects of Insulin Suppression," *Int. J. Obesity* 28 (2004): 1344–48.

16 R. H. Lustig, "Childhood Obesity: Behavioral Aberration or Biochemical Drive? Reinterpreting the First Law of Thermodynamics," *Nature Clin. Pract. Endo. Metab.* 2 (2006): 447–58.

17 M. Kellerer et al., "Insulin Inhibits Leptin Receptor Signalling in HEK293 Cells at the Level of Janus Kinase-2: a Potential Mechanism for Hyperinsulinaemia-

Associated Leptin Resistance," *Diabetologia* 44 (2001): 1125–32; J. W. Hill et al., "Acute Effects of Leptin Require PI3K Signaling in Hypothalamic Proopiomelanocortin Neurons in Mice," *J. Clin. Invest.* 118 (2008): 1796–805; T. Klöckener et al., "High-fat Feeding Promotes Obesity via Insulin Receptor/ PI3K-Dependent Inhibition of SF-1 VMH Neurons," *Nat. Neurosci.* 14 (2001): 911–18.

18   V. D. Castracane et al., "Serum Leptin in Nonpregnant and Pregnant Women and in Old and New World Nonhuman Primates," *Exp. Biol. Med.* 230 (2005): 251–54.

19   Lustig, "Childhood Obesity," pp. 447–58.

Chapter 5

1   K. D. Carr et al., "Evidence of Increased Dopamine Receptor Signaling in Food-Restricted Rats," *Neuroscience* 119 (2003): 1157–67.

2   M. L. Pelchat, "Of Human Bondage: Food Craving, Obsession, Compulsion, and Addiction," *Physiol. Behav.* 76, (2002): 347–52.

3   I. S. Farooqi et al., "Leptin Regulates Striatal Regions and Human Eating Behavior," *Science* epub, August 9, 2007/science.1144599 (2007).

4   L. Carvelli et al., "PI3-Kinase Regulation of Dopamine Uptake," *J. Neurochem.* 81 (2002): 859–69.

5   E. Anderzhanova et al., "Altered Basal and Stimulated Accumbens Dopamine Release in Obese OLETF Rats as a Function of Age and Diabetic Status," *Am. J. Physiol. Regul. Integr. Comp. Physiol.* 293 (2007): R603–R11.

6   K. C. Berridge, "'Liking' and 'Wanting' Food Rewards: Brain Substrates and Roles in Eating Disorders," *Physiol. Behav.* 97 (2009): 537–50.

7   A. K. Garber et al., "Is Fast Food Addictive?" *Curr. Drug Abuse Rev.* 4 (2011): 146–62.

8   T. Dumanovsky et al., "What People Buy from Fast-Food Restaurants: Caloric Content and Menu Item Selection, New York City 2007," *Obesity* 17 (2007): 1369–74.

9   R. D. Mattes, "The Taste for Salt in Humans," *Am. J. Clin. Nutr.* 65 (1997): 692S–97S.

10   A. Drewnowski et al., "Cream and Sugar: Human Preferences for High-Fat Foods," *Physiol. Behav.* 30 (1983): 629–33.

11   G. A. Bernstein et al., "Caffeine Withdrawal in Normal School-Age Children," *J. Am. Acad. Child Adolesc. Psychiatry* 37 (1998): 858–65.

12   C. Huang et al., "Calories from Beverages Purchased at 2 Major Coffee Chains in New York City, 2007," *Prev. Chronic Dis.* 6 (2009): A118.

13   L. R. Vartanian et al., "Effects of Soft Drink Consumption on Nutrition and Health: A Systematic Review and Meta-Analysis," *Am. J. Public Health* 97 (2007): 667–75.

14   N. M. Avena et al., "Evidence for Sugar Addiction: Behavioral and

Neurochemical Effects of Intermittent, Excessive Sugar Intake," *Neurosci. Biobehav. Rev.* 32 (2008): 20–39.

15 M. L. Kringelbach et al., "The Functional Neuroanatomy of Pleasure and Happiness," *Discov. Med.* 9 (2010): 579–87.

16 L. Christensen et al., "Changing Food Preference as a Function of Mood," *J. Psychol.* 140 (2006): 293–306.

17 Can food really be addictive? Yes, says a national drug expert. See http://healthland.time.com/2012/04/05/yes-food-can-be-addictive-says-the-director-of-the-national-institute-on-drug-abuse/.

18 H. Ziauddeen et al., "Obesity and the Brain: How Convincing Is the Addiction Model?" *Nature Rev. Neurosci.* 13 (2012): 279–86.

19 M. E. Bocarsly et al., "Effects of Perinatal Exposure to Palatable Diets on Body Weight and Sensitivity to Drugs of Abuse in Rats," *Physiol. Behav.* (2012) epub May 4, doi:10.1016/j.physbeh.2012.04.024.

Chapter 6

1   B. M. Kudielka et al., "Human Models in Acute and Chronic Stress: Assessing Determinants of Individual Hypothalamus-Pituitary-Adrenal Axis Activity and Reactivity," *Stress* 13 (2010): 1–14.

2   P. Bjorntorp, "Do Stress Reactions Cause Abdominal Obesity and Comorbidities?" *Obes. Rev.* 2 (2001): 73–86.

3   P. A. Tataranni et al., "Effects of Glucocorticoids on Energy Metabolism and Food Intake in Humans," *Am. J. Physiol.* 271 (1996): E317–E25.

4   M. Elovainio et al., "Socioeconomic Differences in Cardiometabolic Factors: Social Causation or Health-Related Selection? Evidence from the Whitehall II Cohort Study, 1991–2004," *Am. J. Epidemiol.* 174 (2011): 779–89.

5   J. P. Shonkoff et al., "Neuroscience, Molecular Biology, and the Childhood Roots of Health Disparities: Building a New Framework for Health Promotion and Disease Prevention," *JAMA* 301 (2009): 2252–59.

6   R. M. Sapolsky, "Depression, Antidepressants, and the Shrinking Hippocampus," *Proc. Natl. Acad. Sci.* 98 (2001): 12320–22.

7   M. F. Dallman et al., "Chronic Stress and Comfort Foods: Self-Medication and Abdominal Obesity," *Brain Behav. Immun.* 19 (2005): 275–80.

8   A. J. Tomiyama et al., "Comfort Food Is Comforting to Those Most Stressed: Evidence of the Chronic Stress Response Network in High Stress Women," *Psychoneuroendocrinology* 36 (2011): 1513–19.

9   A. Sadeh et al., "Sleep Patterns and Sleep Disruptions in School-Age Children," *Dev. Psychol.* 36 (2000): 291–301.

10 C. Benedict et al., "Acute Sleep Deprivation Enhances the Brain's Response to Hedonic Food Stimuli: An fMRI Study," *J. Clin. Endocr. Metab.* 97 (2012): E443–47.

11 D. Kaufman et al., "Early-Life Stress and the Development of Obesity and Insulin Resistance in Juvenile Bonnet Macaques," *Diabetes* 56 (2007): 1382–86.

12   J. P. Warne et al., "Disengaging Insulin from Corticosterone: Roles of Each on Energy Intake and Disposition," *Am. J. Physiol. Reg. Integ. Comp. Physiol.* 296 (2009): R1366–R75.

13   M. L. Mietus-Snyder et al., "Childhood Obesity: Adrift in the "Limbic Triangle," *Ann. Rev. Med.* 59 (2008): 119–34.

Chapter 7

1   K. L. Spalding et al., "Dynamics of Fat Cell Turnover in Humans," *Nature* 453 (2008): 783–87.

2   R. L. Bergmann et al., "Secular Trends in Neonatal Macrosomia in Berlin: Influences of Potential Determinants," *Paediatr. Perinat. Epidemiol.* 17 (2003): 244–49.

3   D. S. Ludwig et al., "The Association Between Pregnancy Weight Gain and Birth Weight: A Within Family Comparison," *Lancet* 376 (2010): 984–90.

4   R. C. Huang et al., "Sex Dimorphism in the Relation Between Early Adiposity and Cardiometabolic Risk in Adolescents," *J. Clin. Endocr. Metab.* 97 (2012): E1014–22.

5   R. J. F. Loos et al., "Genome-wide Association Studies and Human Population Obesity," in *Obesity Before Birth*, R. H. Lustig ed. (New York: Springer, 2010), pp. 95–112.

6   K. M. Godfrey et al., "Epigenetic Gene Promoter Methylation at Birth Is Associated with Child's Later Adiposity," *Diabetes* 60 (2011): 1528–34.

7   D. J. Barker, "The Developmental Origins of Chronic Adult Disease," *Acta Paediatr. Supp.* 93 (2004): 26–33.

8   T. J. Roseboom et al., "Effects of Prenatal Exposure to the Dutch Famine on Adult Disease in Later Life: An Overview," *Mol. Cell. Endocrinol.* 185 (2001): 93–98.

9   C. S. Yajnik et al., "Adiposity and Hyperinsulnemia in Indians Are Present at Birth," *J. Clin. Endocr. Metab.* 87 (2002): 5575–80.

10   P. L. Hofman et al., "Premature birth and Later Insulin Resistance," *N. Engl. J. Med.* 351 (2004): 2179–86.

11   C. M. Boney et al., "Metabolic Syndrome in Childhood: Association with Birth Weight, Maternal Obesity, and Gestational Diabetes," *Pediatrics* 115 (2005): e290–e96.

12   S. G. Bouret et al., "Trophic Action of Leptin on Hypothalamic Neurons That Regulate Feeding," *Science* 304 (2004): 108–10.

13   B. A. Swinburn et al., "Estimating the Changes in Energy Flux That Characterize the Rise in Obesity Prevalence," *Am. J. Clin. Nutr.* 89 (2009): 1723–28.

14   N. A. Christakis et al., "The Spread of Obesity in a Large Social Network over 32 Years," *N. Engl. J. Med.* 357 (2007): 370–79.

15   A. L. Rosenbloom et al., "Age-Adjusted Analysis of Insulin Responses During Normal and Abnormal Glucose Tolerance Tests in Children and Adolescents," *Diabetes* 24 (1975): 820–28.

16   B. E. Corkey, "Banting Lecture 2011: Hyperinsulinemia: Cause or
     Consequence?" *Diabetes* 61 (2012): 4–13.

Chapter 8

1   Y. W. Park et al., "The Metabolic Syndrome: Prevalence and Associated Risk
     Factor Findings in the US Population from the Third National Health and
     Nutrition Examination Survey, 1988–1994," *Arch. Intern. Med.* 163 (2003):
     427–36.
2   E. E. Calle et al., "Obesity and Mortality," *N. Engl. J. Med.* 353 (2005): 2197–99.
3   A. Garg, "Clinical Review: Lipodystrophies: Genetic and Acquired Body Fat
     Disorders," *J. Clin. Endocr. Metab.* 96 (2011): 3313–25.
4   R. Huxley et al., "Body Mass Index, Waist Circumference and Waist:Hip Ratio as
     Predictors of Cardiovascular Risk: A Review of the Literature," *Eur. J. Clin.
     Nutr.* 64 (2010): 16–22.
5   N. R. Shah et al., "Measuring Adiposity in Patients: The Utility of Body Mass
     Index (BMI), Percent Body Fat, and Leptin," PLoS One 10.1371/journal.
     pone.0033308 (2012).
6   E. L. Thomas et al., "The Missing Risk: MRI and MRS Phenotyping of
     Abdominal Adiposity and Ectopic Fat," *Obesity* 20 (2012): 76–87.
7   M. A. Elobeid et al., "Waist Circumference Values Are Increasing Beyond Those
     Expected from BMI Increases," *Obesity* 15 (2007): 2380–83.
8   E. J. Jacobs et al., "Waist Circumference and All-Cause Mortality in a Large US
     Cohort," *Arch. Int. Med.* 170 (2010): 1293–301.
9   M. Khoury et al., "Role of Waist Measures in Characterizing the Lipid and Blood
     Pressure Assessment of Adolescents Classified by Body Mass Index," *Arch.
     Pediatr. Adolesc. Med.* (2012), DOI: 10.1001/archpediatrics.2012.126.
10   B. S. Mohammed et al., "Long-Term Effects of Large-Volume Liposuction on
     Metabolic Risk Factors for Coronary Heart Disease," *Obesity* 16 (2008): 2648–
     51.
11   F. Magkos et al., "Management of the Metabolic Syndrome and Type 2 Diabetes
     Through Lifestyle Modification," *Ann. Rev. Nutr.* 29 (2009): 223–56.

Chapter 9

1   K. R. Fontaine et al., "Years of Life Lost Due to Obesity," *JAMA* 289 (2003): 187–
     93.
2   E. Kassi et al., "Metabolic Syndrome: Definitions and Controversies," *BMC Med.*
     9 (2011): 48.
3   J. Steinberger et al., "Progress and Challenges in Metabolic Syndrome in
     Children and Adolescents: A Scientific Statement from the American Heart
     Association Atherosclerosis, Hypertension, and Obesity in the Young
     Committee of the Council on Cardiovascular Disease in the Young; Council on

Cardiovascular Nursing; and Council on Nutrition, Physical Activity, and Metabolism," *Circulation* 119 (2009): 628–47.

4   A. A. Bremer et al., "State of the Art: Toward a Unifying Hypothesis of Metabolic Syndrome," *Pediatrics* 129 (2012): 557–70.

5   Ibid.

6   A. J. Lusis et al., "Metabolic Syndrome: From Epidemiology to Systems Biology," *Nat. Rev. Genet.* 9 (2008): 819–30.

7   A. A. Bremer et al., "State of the Art: Toward a Unifying Hypothesis of Metabolic Syndrome," *Pediatrics* 129 (2012): 557–70.

8   L. H. Tetri et al., "Severe NAFLD with Hepatic Necroinflammatory Changes in Mice Fed Trans Fats and a High-Fructose Corn Syrup Equivalent," *Am. J. Physiol. Gastrointest. Liver Physiol.* 295 (2008): G987–G95.

9   C. B. Newgard et al., "A Branched-Chain Amino Acid-Related Metabolic Signature That Differentiates Obese and Lean Humans and Contributes to Insulin Resistance," *Cell Metab.* 9 (2009): 311–26.

10   A. Di Castelnuovo et al., "Alcohol Consumption and Cardiovascular Risk: Mechanisms of Action and Epidemiologic Perspectives," *Future Cardiol.* 5 (2009): 467–77.

11   Y. Sakurai et al., "Relation of Total and Beverage-Specific Alcohol Intake to Body Mass Index and Waist-to-Hip Ratio: A Study of Self-Defense Officials in Japan," *Eur. J. Epidemiol.* 13 (1997): 893–98; I. Baik et al., "Prospective Study of Alcohol Consumption and Metabolic Syndrome," *Am. J. Clin. Nutr.* 87 (2008): 1455–63.

12   S. Rahangdale et al., "Therapeutic Interventions and Oxidative Stress in Diabetes," *Front. Biosci.* 14 (2009): 192–209.

Chapter 10

1   G. D. Foster et al., "A Randomized Trial of a Low-Carbohydrate Diet for Obesity," *N. Engl. J. Med.* 348 (2003): 2082–90; F. F. Samaha et al., "A Low-Carbohydrate as Compared with a Low-Fat Diet in Severe Obesity," *N. Engl. J. Med.* 348 (May 22, 2003): 2074–81, at 10.1056/NEJMoa022637348/21/2074.

2   S. R. Smith, "A Look at the Low-Carbohydrate Diet," *N. Engl. J. Med.* 361 (2008): 2286–88.

3   G. E. Fraser, "Vegetarian Diets: What Do We Know of Their Effects on Common Chronic Diseases?" *Am. J. Clin. Nutr.* 89 (2009): 1607S–12S.

4   P. Hujoel, "Dietary Carbohydrats and Dental-Systemic Diseases," *Crit. Rev. Oral Biol. Med.* 88 (2009): 490–502.

5   M. S. Brown et al., "A Receptor-Mediated Pathway for Cholesterol Homeostasis," *Science* 232 (1986): 34–47.

6   G. Taubes, "Nutrition: The Soft Science of Dietary Fat," *Science* 291 (2001): 2536–45.

7   P. W. Siri-Tarino et al., "Saturated Fat, Carbohydrate, and Cardiovascular Disease," *Am. J. Clin. Nutr.* 91 (2010): 502–9.

8   A. Astrup et al., "The Role of Reducing Intakes of Saturated Fat in the
    Prevention of Cardiovascular Disease: Where Does the Evidence Stand in
    2010?" *Am. J. Clin. Nutr.* 93 (2011): 684–88.
9   B. V. Howard et al., "Low-Fat Dietary Pattern and Risk of Cardiovascular
    Disease: The Women's Health Initiative Randomized Controlled Dietary
    Modification Trial," *JAMA* 295 (2006): 655–66; B. V. Howard et al., "Low-Fat
    Dietary Pattern and Weight Change over 7 Years: The Women's Health Initiative
    Dietary Modification Trial," *JAMA* 295 (2006): 39–49.
10 A. Accurso et al., "Dietary Carbohydrate Reduction in Type 2 Diabetes Mellitus
    and Metabolic Syndrome: A Critical Re-Appraisal," *Nutr. Metab. (Lond)* 5
    (2008): 9.

Chapter 11

1   M. B. Vos et al., "Dietary Fructose Consumption Among US Children and
    Adults: The Third National Health and Nutrition Examination Survey,"
    Medscape J. Med. 10, (2008): 160.
2   Sugar and Sweeteners Team Market and Trade Economics, Economic Research
    Service, U.S. Dept. Of Agriculture, U.S. Per Capita Caloric Sweeteners Estimated
    Deliveries for Domestic Food and Beverage Use, by Calendar Year (2010), www
    .ers.usda.gov/briefing/Sugar/data/table50.xls.
3   R. K. Johnson et al., "Dietary Sugars Intake and Cardiovascular Health: A
    Scientific Statement from the American Heart Association," *Circulation* 120
    (2009): 1011–20.
4   Ibid.
5   R. H. Lustig et al., "The Toxic Truth about Sugar," *Nature* 487 (2012): 27–29.
6   M. T. Le et al., "Effects of High-Fructose Corn Syrup and Sucrose on the
    Pharmacokinetics of Fructose and Acute Metabolic and Hemodynamic
    Responses in Healthy Subjects," *Metabolism* 61 (2012): 641–51.
7   R. H. Lustig, "Fructose: Metabolic, Hedonic, and Societal Parallels with
    Ethanol," *J. Am. Diet. Assoc.* 110 (2010): 1307–21.
8   W. L. Dills, "Protein Fructosylation: Fructose and the Maillard Reaction," *Am. J.
    Clin. Nutr.* 58 (1993): 779S–87S.
9   V. T. Samuel, "Fructose Induced Lipogenesis: From Sugar to Fat to Insulin
    Resistance," *Trends Endocrinol. Metab.* 22 (2011): 60–65.
10 R. J. Shaw et al., "Decoding Key Nodes in the Metabolism of Cancer Cells: Sugar
    and Spice and All Things Nice," *F1000 Biol. Rep.* 4 (2012): 2.
11 S. Thuy et al., "Nonalcoholic Fatty Liver Disease in Humans Is Associated with
    Increased Plasma Endotoxin and Plasminogen Activator Inhibitor 1
    Concentrations and with Fructose Intake," *J. Nutr.* 138 (2008): 1452–55.
12 M. Maersk et al., "Sucrose-Sweetened Beverages Increase Fat Storage in the
    Liver, Muscle, and Visceral Fat Depot: A 6-Mo Randomized Intervention Study,"
    Am. J. Clin. Nutr. 95 (2012): 283–89; N. K. Pollock et al., "Greater Fructose

Consumption Is Associated with Cardiometabolic Risk Markers and Visceral Adiposity in Adolescents," *J. Nutr.* 142 (2012): 251–57.

13 R. S. O'Shea et al., "Alcoholic Liver Disease," *Am. J. Gastroenterol.* 105 (2010): 14–32.

14 C. D. Knott, "Changes in Orangutan Caloric Intake, Energy Balance, and Ketones in Response to Fluctuating Fruit Availability," *Int. J. Primatol.* 19 (1998): 1061–79.

Chapter 12

1 J. J. Otten et al., "Dietary Reference Intakes: The Essential Guide to Nutrient Requirements," National Academy of Sciences, 2006.

2 J. D. Leach, "Evolutionary Perspective on Dietary Intake of Fibre and Colorectal Cancer," *Eur. J. Clin. Nutr.* 61 (2007): 140–42.

3 M. O. Weickert et al., "Metabolic Effects of Dietary Fiber Consumption and Prevention of Diabetes," *J. Nutr.* 138 (2008): 439–42.

4 R. E. Post et al., "Dietary Fiber for the Treatment of Type 2 Diabetes Mellitus," *J. Am. Board Fam. Med.* 25 (2012): 16–23.

5 R. Levine, "Monosaccharides in Health and Disease," *Ann. Rev. Nutr.* 6 (1986): 211–24.

6 C. J. Small et al., "Gut Hormones and the Control of Appetite," *Trends Endocrinol. Metab.* 15 (2004): 259–63.

7 P. D. Cani et al., "Gut Microbiota Fermentation of Prebiotics Increases Satietogenic and Incretin Gutpeptide Production with Consequences for Appetite Sensation and Glucose Response after a Meal," *Am. J. Clin. Nutr.* 90 (2009): 1236–43.

8 D. Lairon et al., "Digestible and Indigestible Carbohydrates: Interactions with Postprandial Lipid Metabolism," *J. Nutr. Biochem.* 18 (2007): 217–27.

9 G. D. Brinkworth et al., "Comparative Effects of Very Low-Carbohydrate, High-Fat and High-Carbohydrate, Low-Fat Weight-Loss Diets on Bowel Habit and Faecal Short-Chain Fatty Acids and Bacterial Populations," *Br. J. Nutr.* 101, 1493–502.

10 R. Krajmalnik-Brown et al., "Effects of Gut Microbes on Nutrient Absorption and Energy Regulation," *Nutr. Clin. Pract.* 27 (2012): 201–14.

11 G. D. Wu et al., "Linking Long-Term Dietary Patterns with Gut Microbial Enterotypes," *Science* 334 (2011): 105–8.

12 A. D. Liese et al., "Dietary Glycemic Index and Glycemic Load, Carbohydrate and Fiber Intake, and Measures of Insulin Sensitivity, Secretion, and Adiposity in the Insulin Resistance Atherosclerosis Study," *Diab. Care* 28 (2005): 2832–38.

13 M. B. Schulze et al., "Fiber and Magnesium Intake and Incidence of Type 2 Diabetes: A Prospective Study and Meta-Analysis," *Arch. Int. Med.* 167 (2007): 956–65.

14 J. S. De Munter et al., "Whole Grain, Bran, and Germ Intake and Risk of Type 2

Diabetes: A Prospective Cohort Study and Systematic Review," *PLoS Med.* 4 (2007): e261.

Chapter 13

1   K. Shaw et al., "Exercise for Overweight or Obesity," Cochrane Database Syst. Rev. CD003817 (2006).
2   K. D. Hall et al., "Quantification of the Effect of Energy Imbalance on Bodyweight," *Lancet* 378 (2011): 826–37.
3   R. L. Leibel et al., "Changes in Energy Expenditure Resulting from Altered Body Weight," *N. Engl. J. Med.* 332 (1995): 621–28.
4   M. T. Bekx et al., "Decreased Energy Expenditure Is Caused by Abnormal Body Composition in Infants with Prader-Willi Syndrome," *J. Pediatr.* 143 (2003): 372–76.
5   K. J. Acheson et al., "Protein Choices Targeting Thermogenesis and Metabolism," *Am. J. Clin. Nutr.* 93 (2011): 525–34.
6   D. S. Ludwig, "The Glycemic Index: Physiological Mechanisms Relating to Obesity, Diabetes, and Cardiovascular Disease," *JAMA* 287 (2002): 2414–23.
7   J. A. Mitchell et al., "The Impact of Combined Health Factors on Cardiovascular Disease Mortality," *Am. Heart J.* 160 (2010): 102–8.
8   C. P. Wen et al., "Minimum Amount of Physical Activity for Reduced Mortality and Extended Life Expectancy: A Prospective Cohort Study," *Lancet* 378 (2011): 1244–53.
9   J. P. Little et al., "Skeletal Muscle and Beyond: The Role of Exercise as a Mediator of Systemic Mitochondrial Biogenesis," *Appl. Physiol. Nutr. Metab.* 36 (2011): 598–607.
10 V. Teixeira et al., "Antioxidant Status, Oxidative Stress, and Damage in Elite Kayakers After 1 Year of Training and Competition in 2 Seasons," *Appl. Physiol. Nutr. Metab.* 34 (2009): 716–24.
11 J. L. Glick, "Effects of Exercise on Oxidative Activities in Rat Liver Mitochondria," *Am. J. Physiol.* 210 (1966): 1215–21.
12 M. J. Gibala et al., "Physiological Adaptations to Low-Volume, High-Intensity Interval Training in Health and Disease," *J. Physiol.* 590, no. 5 (2012): 1077–84.
13 D. Stensvold et al., "Strength Training versus Aerobic Interval Training to Modify Risk Factors of Metabolic Syndrome," *J. Appl. Physiol.* 108 (2010): 804–10.
14 K. Manias et al., "Fractures and Recurrent Fractures in Children; Varying Effects of Environmental Factors as Well as Bone Size and Mass," *Bone* 39 (2006): 652–57.
15 S. Bajpeyi et al., "Effect of Exercise Intensity and Volume on Persistence of Insulin Sensitivity During Training Cessation," *J. Appl. Physiol.* 106 (2009): 1079–85.
16 G. P. Nassis et al., "Central and Total Adiposity Are Lower in Overweight and

Obese Children with High Cardiorespiratory Fitness," *Eur. J. Clin. Nutr.* 59 (2005): 137–41.

17 C. Padilla-Moledo et al., "Cardiorespiratory Fitness and Fatness Are Associated with Health Complaints and Health Risk Behaviors in Youth," *J. Phys. Act. Health* epub, July 29, 2011.

18 P. A. McAuley et al., "Obesity Paradox and Cardiorespiratory Fitness in 12,417 Male Veterans Aged 40 to 70 Years," *Mayo Clin. Proc.* 85 (2010): 115–21.

19 E. E. Calle et al., "Obesity and Mortality," *N. Engl. J. Med.* 353 (2005): 2197–99.

Chapter 14

1 G. Davì et al., "Nutraceuticals in Diabetes and Metabolic Syndrome," *Cardiovasc. Ther.* 28 (2010): 216–26.

2 P. T. Gee, "Unleashing the Untold and Misunderstood Observations on Vitamin E," *Genes Nutr.* 6 (2011): 5–16.

3 C. S. Maxwell et al., "Update on Vitamin D and Type 2 Diabetes," *Nutr. Rev.* 69 (2011): 291–95.

4 O. Vang et al., "What Is New for an Old Molecule? Systematic Review and Recommendations on the Use of Resveratrol," *PLoS One* 6 (2011): e19881.

5 J. Mursu et al., "Dietary Supplements and Mortality Rate in Older Women: The Iowa Women's Health Study," *Arch. Int. Med.* 171 (2011): 1625–33.

6 G. Bjelakovic et al., "Antioxidant Supplements for Prevention of Mortality in Healthy Participants and Patients with Various Diseases," *Cochrane Database Syst. Rev.* 3:CD007176 (2012).

Chapter 15

1 E. Weil, "Puberty Before Age 10: A New 'Normal'?" *New York Times Magazine*, March 30, 2012, www.nytimes.com/2012/04/01/magazine/puberty-before-age-10-a-new-normal.html?pagewanted=all.

2 F. M. Biro et al., "Pubertal Assessment Method and Baseline Characteristics in a Mixed Longitudinal Study of Girls," *Pediatrics* 126 (2010): e583–e90.

3 H. S. Mumby et al., "Mendelian Randomisation Study of Childhood BMI and Early Menarche," *J. Obes.* (2011): 180729.

4 C. B. Jasik et al., "Adolescent Obesity and Puberty: The 'Perfect Storm,'" *Ann. NY. Acad. Sci.* 1135 (2008): 265–79.

5 S. L. Verhulst et al., "Intrauterine Exposure to Environmental Pollutants and Body Mass Index During the First 3 Years of Life," *Environ. Health Perspect.* 117 (2009): 122–26.

6 J. L. Carwile et al., "Urinary Bisphenol A and Obesity: NHANES 2003–2006," *Environ. Res.* 111 (2011): 825–30.

7 S. L. Teitelbaum et al., "Associations Between Phthalate Metabolite Urinary

Concentrations and Body Size Measures in New York City Children," *Environ. Res.* 112 (2012): 186–93.

8   M. Carfi et al., "TBTC Induces Adipocyte Differentiation in Human Bone Marrow Long Term Culture," *Toxicology* 249 (2008): 11–18.

9   M. Jerrett et al., "Automobile Traffic Around the Home and Attained Body Mass Index: A Longitudinal Cohort Study of Children Aged 10–18 Years," *Prev. Med.* 50 Suppl. 1 (2010): S50–S58.

10   C. Gabbert et al., "Adenovirus 36 and Obesity in Children and Adolescents," *Pediatrics* 126 (2010): 721–26.

11   Y. C. Klimentidis et al., "Canaries in the Coal Mine: A Cross-Species Analysis of the Plurality of Obesity Epidemics," *Proc. Biol. Sci.* 278 (2011): 1626–32.

Chapter 16

1   R. K. Johnson et al., "Dietary Sugars Intake and Cardiovascular Health: A Scientific Statement from the American Heart Association," *Circulation* 120 (2009): 1011–20.

2   U.S. Senate, "Dietary Goals for the United States," 95th Congress, U.S. Government Printing Office, Washington, D.C., 1977.

3   U.S. Department of Agriculture, Economic Research Service, Sugar and Sweeteners: Background. Washington, D.C., 2011.

4   W. L. Dills, "Protein Fructosylation: Fructose and the Maillard Reaction," *Am. J. Clin. Nutr.* 58 (1993): 779S–87S.

5   D. Gonsolin et al., "High Dietary Sucrose Triggers Hyperinsulinemia, Increases Myocardial B-Oxidation, Reduces Glycolytic Flux, And Delays Post-Ischemic Contractile Recovery," *Mol. Cell. Biochem.* 295 (2007): 217–28.

6   G. Livesey, "Fructose Ingestion: Dose-Dependent Responses in Health Research," *J. Nutr.* 139 (2009): 1246S–52S.

7   J. J. Rumessen et al., "Absorption Capacity of Fructose in Healthy Adults: Comparison with Sucrose and Its Constituent Monosaccharides," *Gut* 27 (1986): 1161–68.

8   M. Takeuchi et al., "Immunological Detection of Fructose-Derived Advanced Glycation End-Products," *Lab Invest.* 90 (2010): 1117–27.

9   M. K. Pickens et al., "Dietary Sucrose Is Essential to the Development of Liver Injury in the MCD Model of Steatohepatitis," *J. Lipid Res.* 50 (2009): 2072–82.

10   J. L. Sievenpiper et al., "Effect of Fructose on Body Weight in Controlled Feeding Trials: A Systematic Review and Meta-Analysis," *Ann. Int. Med.* 156 (2012): 291–304.

11   E. J. Parks et al., "Effects of a Low-Fat, High-Carbohydrate Diet on VLDL-Triglyceride Assembly, Production, and Clearance," *J. Clin. Invest.* 104 (1999): 1087–96.

12   101st Congress, HR 3562, Nutrition Labeling and Education Act, U.S.

Government Printing Office, 1990, thomas.loc.gov/cgi-bin/bdquery/
z?d101:H.R.3562.

13 J. L. Harris et al., "Fast Food FACTS: Evaluating Fast Food Nutrition and
    Marketing to Youth," Rudd Center for Food Policy and Obesity, 2010), at
    fastfoodmarketing.org/.

14 L. Gómez et al., "Sponsorship of Physical Activity Programs by the Sweetened
    Beverages Industry: Public Health or Public Relations?" *Rev. Saude Publica* 45
    (2011): 423–27.

Chapter 17

1   E. Isganaitis et al., "Fast Food, Central Nervous System Insulin Resistance, and
    Obesity," *Arterioscler. Thromb. Vasc. Biol.* 25 (2005): 2451–62.

2   B. Sjouke et al., "Familial Hypercholesterolemia: Present and Future
    Management," *Curr. Cardiol. Rep.* 13 (2011): 527–36.

3   R. M. Krauss, "Atherogenic Lipoprotein Phenotype and Diet-Gene Interactions,"
    J. Nutr. 131 (2001): 340S–43S.

4   I. Aeberli et al., "Fructose Intake Is a Predictor of LDL Particle Size in
    Overweight Schoolchildren," *Am. J. Clin. Nutr.* 86 (2007): 1174–78.

5   A. Accurso et al., "Dietary Carbohydrate Reduction in Type 2 Diabetes Mellitus
    and Metabolic Syndrome. A Critical Re-Appraisal," *Nutr. Metab. (Lond)* 5
    (2008): 9.

6   S. Y. Foo et al., "Vascular Effects of a Low-Carbohydrate High-Protein Diet,"
    Proc. Natl. Acad. Sci. 106 (2009): 15418–23.

7   C. D. Gardner et al., "Micronutrient Quality of Weight-Loss Diets That Focus on
    Macronutrients: Results from the A to Z Study," *Am. J. Clin. Nutr.* 92 (2010): 304–12.

8   G. D. Foster et al., "A Randomized Trial of a Low-Carbohydrate Diet for
    Obesity," *N. Engl. J. Med.* 348 (2003): 2082–90; F. F. Samaha et al., "A Low-
    Carbohydrate as Compared with a Low-Fat Diet in Severe Obesity," *N. Engl. J.
    Med.* 348 (May 22, 2003): 2074–81, 10.1056/NEJMoa022637348/21/2074.

9   U. Lindmark et al., "Food Selection Associated with Sense of Coherence in
    Adults," *Nutr. J.* 4 (2005): 9 (2005), 10.1186/1475-2891-4-9.

10 M. Bulló et al., "Mediterranean Diet and Oxidation: Nuts and Olive Oil as
    Important Sources of Fat and Antioxidants," *Curr. Top. Med. Chem.* 11 (2011):
    1797–810.

11 D. Ornish et al., "Increased Telomerase Activity and Comprehensive Lifestyle
    Changes: A Pilot Study," *Lancet Oncol.* 9 (2008): 1048–57.

12 C. D. Gardner et al., "Comparison of the Atkins, Zone, Ornish, and LEARN
    Diets for Change in Weight and Related Risk Factors Among Overweight
    Premenopausal Women: The A to Z Weight Loss Study: A Randomized Trial,"
    JAMA 298 (2007): 969–77.

13 S. B. Eaton et al., "Paleolithic Nutrition: A Consideration of Its Nature and
    Current Implications," *N. Engl. J. Med.* 312 (1985): 283–89.

14   S. Lindeberg, "Palaeolithic Diet ('Stone Age' Diet)," *Scand. J. Food Nutr.* 49 (2005): 75–77.

15   L. A. Frassetto et al., "Metabolic and Physiologic Improvements from Consuming a Paleolithic, Hunter-Gatherer Type Diet," *Eur. J. Clin. Nutr.* 63 (2009): 947–55.

16   D. S. Ludwig, "The Glycemic Index: Physiological Mechanisms Relating to Obesity, Diabetes, and Cardiovascular Disease," *JAMA* 287 (2002): 2414–23.

17   A. Esfahani et al., "The Application of the Glycemic Index and Glycemic Load in Weight Loss: A Review of the Clinical Evidence," *IUBMB Life* 63 (2011): 7–13.

18   C. B. Ebbeling et al., "Effects of a Low-Glycemic Load vs Low-Fat Diet in Obese Young Adults: A Randomized Trial," *JAMA* 297 (2007): 2092–102.

19   M. D. Nelson et al., "Genotype Patterns Predict Weight Loss Success: The Right Diet Does Matter," Cardiovascular Disease Epidemiology and Prevention and Nutrition, Physical Activity, and Metabolism San Francisco, CA (abstract), 2010, www.theheart.org/article/1053429.do.

20   Ebbeling et al., "Effects of a Low-Glycemic Load vs Low-Fat Diet," pp. 2092–102.

21   Gardner et al., "Comparison of the Atkins, Zone, Ornish, and LEARN Diets," pp. 969–77; M. A. Cornier et al., "Insulin Sensitivity Determines the Effectiveness of Dietary Macronutrient Composition on Weight Loss in Obese Women," *Obesity Res.* 13 (2005): 703–9.

22   Q. Qi et al., "Insulin Receptor Substrate 1 Gene Variation Modifies Insulin Resistance Response to Weight-Loss Diets in a 2-Year Randomized Trial: The Preventing Overweight Using Novel Dietary Strategies (Pounds Lost) Trial," *Circulation* 124 (2011): 563–71.

23   R. Dhingra et al., "Soft Drink Consumption and Risk of Developing Cardiometabolic Risk Factors and the Metabolic Syndrome in Middle-Aged Adults in the Community," *Circulation* 116 (2007): 480–88.

24   M. Y. Pepino et al., "Non-Nutritive Sweeteners, Energy Balance, and Glucose Homeostasis," *Curr. Opin. Clin. Nutr. Metab. Care* 14 (2011): 391–95.

25   C. Gardner et al., "Nonnutritive Sweeteners: Current Use and Health Perspectives," *Circulation* 126 (2012): 509–19.

26   S. A. Bowman et al., "Effects of Fast-Food Consumption on Energy Intake and Diet Quality Among Children in a National Household Survey," *Pediatrics* 113 (2004): 112–18.

27   California Center for Public Health Advocacy, "Fast Food Nutrition Quiz," Davis, CA, 2007, www.publichealthadvocacy.org/_PDFs/fieldpollresults.pdf.

28   B. J. Rolls et al., "Portion Size of Food Affects Energy Intake in Normal-Weight and Overweight Men and Women," *Am. J. Clin. Nutr.* 76 (2003): 1207–13.

Chapter 18

1   M. S. Faith et al., "Evaluating Parents and Adult Caregivers as 'Agents of Change' for Treating Obese Children: Evidence for Parent Behavior Change Strategies and Research Gaps," *Circulation* 125 (2012): 1186–1207.

2   F. Kreier, "To Be, or Not to Be Obese—That's the Challenge: A Hypothesis on the Cortical Inhibition of the Hypothalamus and Its Therapeutical Consequences," *Med. Hypotheses* 75 (2010): 214–17.

3   J. Bowen et al., "Appetite Hormones and Energy Intake in Obese Men After Consumption of Fructose, Glucose and Whey Protein Beverages," *Int. J. Obes.* 31 (2007): 1696–1703.

4   A. J. Stunkard et al., "Two Forms of Disordered Eating in Obesity: Binge Eating and Night Eating," *Int. J. Obes. Related Met. Disord.* 27 (2003): 1–12.

Chapter 19

1   E. Fabbrini et al., "Intrahepatic Fat, Not Visceral Fat, Is Linked with Metabolic Complications of Obesity," *Proc. Natl. Acad. Sci.* 106 (2009): 15430–35.

2   K. C. Sung et al., "Interrelationship Between Fatty Liver and Insulin Resistance in the Development of Type 2 Diabetes," *J. Clin. Endocrinol. Metab.* 96 (2011): 1093–97.

3   E. Ferrannini et al., "Insulin Resistance and Hypersecretion in Obesity," *J. Clin. Invest.* 100 (1997): 1166–73; C. Preeyasombat et al., "Racial and Etiopathologic Dichotomies in Insulin Secretion and Resistance in Obese Children," *J. Pediatr.* 146 (2005): 474–81.

4   W. H. Herman et al., "Racial and Ethnic Differences in the Relationship Between HbA1c and Blood Glucose: Implications for the Diagnosis of Diabetes," *J. Clin. Endocr. Metab.* epub, January 11, 2012.

5   L. J. Aronne et al., "Emerging Pharmacotherapy for Obesity," *Expert Opin. Emerg. Drugs* 16 (2011): 587–96.

6   A. E. Pontiroli et al., "Long-Term Prevention of Mortality in Morbid Obesity Through Bariatric Surgery: A Systematic Review and Meta-Analysis of Trials Performed with Gastric Banding and Gastric Bypass," *Ann. Surg.* 253 (2011): 484–87.

7   D. S. Zingmond et al., "Hospitalization Before and After Gastric Bypass Surgery," *JAMA* 294 (2005): 1918–24.

8   T. H. Inge et al., "Bariatric Surgery for Overweight Adolescents: Concerns and Recommendations," *Pediatrics* 114 (2004): 217–23.

9   E. C. Mun et al., "Current Status of Medical and Surgical Therapy for Obesity," *Gastroenterology* 120 (2001): 669–81; L. Sjöstrom et al., "Lifestyle, Diabetes, and Cardiovascular Risk Factors 10 Years After Bariatric Surgery," *N. Engl. J. Med.* 351 (2004): 2683–93.

10   M. Shah et al., "Review: Long-Term Impact of Bariatric Surgery on Body Weight, Co-Morbidities, and Nutritional Status," *J. Clin. Endocr. Metab.* 91 (2006): 4223–31.

11   T. J. Hoerger et al., "Cost-Effectiveness of Bariatric Surgery for Severely Obese
     Adults with Diabetes," *Diab. Care* 33 (2010): 1933–39; S. H. Chang et al., "Cost-
     Effectiveness of Bariatric Surgery: Should It Be Universally Available? *Maturitas*
     69 (2011): 230–38.
12   C. Boza et al., "Safety and Efficacy of Roux-en-Y Gastric Bypass to Treat Type 2
     Diabetes Mellitus in Non-Severely Obese Patients," *Obes. Surg.* 21 (2011): 1330–
     36.
13   R. M. Hodson et al., "Management of Obesity with the New Intragastric
     Balloon," *Obes. Surg.* 11 (2001): 327–29.
14   K. Weichman et al., "The Effectiveness of Adjustable Gastric Banding: A
     Retrospective 6-year U.S. Follow-Up Study," *Surg. Endosc.* 25 (2011): 397–403.
15   J. V. Franco et al., "A Review of Studies Comparing Three Laparoscopic
     Procedures in Bariatric Surgery: Sleeve Gastrectomy, Roux-en-Y gastric Bypass
     and Adjustable Gastric Banding," *Obes. Surg.* 21 (2011): 1458–68.
16   M. Michalsky et al., "Developing Criteria for Pediatric/Adolescent Bariatric
     Surgery Programs," *Pediatrics* 128 Supp. 2 (2011): S65–S70.

Chapter 20

1   A. K. Garber et al., "Is Fast Food Addictive?" *Curr. Drug Abuse Rev.* 4 (2011):
     146–62.
2   K. Glanz et al., "How Major Restaurant Chains Plan Their Menus: The Role of
     Profit, Demand, and Health," *Am. J. Prev. Med.* 32 (2007): 383–88.
3   L. Zwirn, "The Recession-Proof Morning Luxury," Boston.com, December 14,
     2011, articles.boston.com/2011-12-14/lifestyle/30516702_1_iced-coffee-coffee-
     drinkers-lattes.
4   Centers for Medicare and Medicaid Services, U.S. Government, 2011. www.cms
     .gov/MedicareMedicaidStatSupp/downloads/2007Table5.5b.pdf.
5   J. Weisenthal, "Medicare to Be Broke by 2024, 5 Years Sooner Than Expected,"
     Business Insider, May 13, 2011 articles.businessinsider.com/2011-05-13/
     news/30082187_1_entitlement medicare-annual-report.

Chapter 21

1   CALPIRG, "Apples to Twinkies: Comparing Federal Subsidies of Fresh Produce
     and Junk Food," 2011, www.calpirg.org/reports/caf/apples-twinkies.
2   W. H. Glinsmann et al., "Evaluation of Health Aspects of Sugars Contained in
     Carbohydrate Sweeteners: Report of Sugars Task Force, 1986," *J. Nutr.* 116
     (1986): 1/S.
3   R. K. Johnson et al., "Dietary Sugars Intake and Cardiovascular Health: A
     Scientific Statement from the American Heart Association," *Circulation* 120
     (2009): 1011–20.
4   Food and Drug Administration, "High Fructose Corn Syrup: Code of Federal

Regulations," U.S. Government Printing Office, Washington, D.C., 1996, vol. 61, pp. 43447, 21CFR 184.1866.

5   R. H. Lustig et al., "The Toxic Truth About Sugar," *Nature* 487 (2012): 27–29.
6   European Food Safety Authority, "Outcome of the Public Consultation on the Draft Opinion of the Scientific Panel on Dietetic Products, Nutrition, and Allergies (NDA) on Dietary Reference Values for Carbohydrates and Dietary Fibre," 2010, www.efsa.europa.eu/en/efsajournal/pub/1508.htm.
7   M. J. Perry, "Sugar Tariffs Cost Americans $2.5 Billion in 2009," 2010, at mjperry.blogspot.com/2010/01/sugar-tariffs-cost-americans-25-billion.html.
8   U.S. Department of Labor, Bureau of Labor Statistics, "Career Guide to Industries, 2010–2011," U.S. Government Printing Office, Washington, D.C., 2011, www.bls.gov/oco/cg/cgs011.htm.
9   World Health Organization, "Diet, Nutrition, and the Prevention of Chronic Diseases," Geneva, 2003, www.who.int/hpr/NPH/docs/who_fao_expert_report.pdf.
10 K. D. Brownell et al., "The Supplemental Nutrition Assistance Program, Soda, and USDA Policy: Who Benefits?" *JAMA* 306 (2011): 1370–71.
11 D. L. Millimet et al., "School Nutrition Programs and the Incidence of Childhood Obesity," *J. Human Resources* 45 (2010): 640–54.
12 M. M. Mello, "Obesity—Personal Choice or Public Health Issue?" *Nature Clin. Pract. Endocrinol. Metab.* 4 (2008): 2–3.
13 H. L. Walls et al., "The Regulatory Gap in Chronic Disease Prevention: A Historical Perspective," *J. Public Health Policy* 33 (2011): 89–104.
14 Federal Trade Commission, "Advertising to Kids and the FTC: A Regulatory Retrospective That Advises the Present," U.S. Government Printing Office, Washington, D.C., 2002, www.ftc.gov/speeches/beales/040802adstokids.pdf.
15 "USDA Role in Food Pyramid Criticized," *Chicago Tribune*, 2003, articles. chicagotribune.com/2003-10-14/news/0310140282_1_dietary-guidelines-usda-food-guide-pyramid.
16 Government Accountability Office, "FDA Should Strengthen Its Oversight of Food Ingredients Determined to be Generally Recognized as Safe (GRAS)," U.S. Government Printing Office, Washington, D.C., 2010, www.gao.gov/assets/310/300753.pdf.

Chapter 22

1   K. Strong et al., "Preventing Chronic Diseases: How Many Lives Can We Save?" *Lancet* 366 (2005): 1578–82.
2   T. Babor et al., *Alcohol: No Ordinary Commodity—Research and Public Policy*, Oxford, UK: Oxford University Press, 2003.
3   R. H. Lustig et al., "The Toxic Truth About Sugar," *Nature* 487 (2012): 27–29.
4   A. I. Patel et al., "Encouraging Consumption of Water in School and Child Care Settings: Access, Challenges, and Strategies for Improvement," *Am. J. Public Health* 101 (2011): 1370–79.

5   R. H. Lustig, "Fructose: Metabolic, Hedonic, and Societal Parallels with
    Ethanol," *J. Am. Diet Assoc.* 110 (2010): 1307–21; J. S. Lim et al., "The Role of
    Fructose in the Pathogenesis of NAFLD and the Metabolic Syndrome," *Nat. Rev.
    Gastroenterol. Hepatol.* 7 (2010): 251–64.

6   N. M. Avena et al., "Evidence for Sugar Addiction: Behavioral and
    Neurochemical Effects of Intermittent, Excessive Sugar Intake," *Neurosci.
    Biobehav. Rev.* 32 (2008): 20–39.

7   A. K. Garber et al., "Is Fast Food Addictive?" *Curr. Drug Abuse Rev.* 4 (2011):
    146–62.

8   E. A. Finkelstein et al., "National Medical Spending Attributable to Overweight
    and Obesity: How Much, and Who's Paying?" *Health Affairs* W3 (2003): 219–26.

9   E. A. Finkelstein et al., "The Costs of Obesity in the Workplace," *J. Occup.
    Environ. Med.* 52 (2010): 971–76.

10 R. Room et al., "Alcohol and Public Health," *Lancet* 365 (2005): 519–30.

11 C. Gonzalez-Suarez et al., "School-Based Interventions on Childhood Obesity:
    A Meta-Analysis," *Am. J. Prev. Med.* 37 (2009): 418–27.

12 H. Saffer, "Alcohol Advertising and Youth," *J. Stud. Alcohol Suppl.* 14 (2002):
    173–81.

13 New York City Department of Health. Man Drinking Fat. www.youtube.com/
    watch?v=-F4t8zL6F0c.

14 T. Dumanovsky et al., "Changes in Energy Content of Lunchtime Purchases
    from Fast Food Restaurants After Introduction of Calorie Labelling: Cross
    Sectional Customer Surveys," *BMJ* (July 26), 343:d4464. doi: 10.1136/bmj
    .d4464.

15 B. Elbel, "Consumer Estimation of Recommended and Actual Calories at Fast
    Food Restaurants," *Obesity* 19 (2011): 1971–78.

16 Environmental Working Group, "Sugar in Children's Cereals," 2011. http://www
    .ewg.org/report/sugar_in_childrens_cereals.

17 K. L. Stanhope et al., "Consuming Fructose-, Not Glucose-Sweetened Beverages
    Increases Visceral Adiposity and Lipids and Decreases Insulin Sensitivity in
    Overweight/Obese Humans," *J. Clin. Invest.* 119 (2009): 1322–34.

18 C. C. Kamath et al., "Clinical Review: Behavioral Interventions to Prevent
    Childhood Obesity: A Systematic Review and Metaanalyses of Randomized
    Trials," *J. Clin. Endocr. Metab.* 93 (2008): 4606–15.

19 L. A. Smith et al., "The Effect of Alcohol Advertising, Marketing and Portrayal
    on Drinking Behaviour in Young People: Systematic Review of Prospective
    Cohort Studies," *BMC Public Health* 9 (2009): 51.

20 T. Babor et al., *Alcohol: No Ordinary Commodity*. Oxford, New York, 2003.

21 Kaiser Family Foundation, "Food for Thought: Television Food Advertising to
    Children in the United States," 2007, www.kff.org/entmedia/upload/7618.pdf.

22 Y. Aktaş Arnas, "The Effects of Television Food Advertisement on Children's
    Food Purchasing Requests," *Pediatr. Int.* 48 (2006): 138–45.

23 R. Koordeman et al., "Exposure to Soda Commercials Affects Sugar-Sweetened

Soda Consumption in Young Women: An Observational Experimental Study," *Appetite* 54 (2010): 619–22.

24 International Association for the Study of Obesity, "Recommendations for an International Code on Marketing of Foods and Non-Alcoholic Beverages to Children," 2007, www.cspinet.org/nutritionpolicy/CI CODE OFFICIAL ENGLISH.pdf.

25 M. C. Jalonick, "Government Pulls Back on Junk Food Marketing Proposal," Salon.com, 2011, www.salon.com/2011/10/12/govt_pulls_back_on_junk_food_marketing_proposal_2/.

26 R. H. Lustig et al., "The Toxic Truth About Sugar," *Nature* 487 (2012): 27–29.

27 D. R. Taber et al., "Banning All Sugar-Sweetened Beverages in Middle Schools: Reduction of In-School Access and Purchasing but Not Overall Consumption," *Arch. Pediatr. Adol. Med.* 166 (2012): 256–62.

28 T. Babor et al., *Alcohol: No Ordinary Commodity*; Room et al., "Alcohol and Public Health," pp. 519–30; L. A. Schmidt et al., "Alcohol: Equity and Social Determinants," in E. Blas et al., *Equity, Social Determinants, and Public Health Programmes,* Geneva, World Health Publications (2010), pp. 11–30.

29 K. D. Brownell et al., "The Public Health and Economic Benefits of Taxing Sugar-Sweetened Beverages," *N. Engl. J. Med.* 361 (2009): 1599–605.

30 G. Woodward-Lopez et al., "To What Extent Have Sweetened Beverages Contributed to the Obesity Epidemic?" *Public Health Nutr.* 23 (2011): 1–11.

31 A. A. Bremer et al., "Effects of Sugar-Sweetened Beverages on Children," *Pediatr. Annals* 41 (2012): 26–30.

32 J. M. Noble et al., "Scurvy and Rickets Masked by Chronic Neurologic Illness: Revisiting 'Psychologic Malnutrition,'" *Pediatrics* 119 (2007): e783–e90.

33 J. M. Fletcher et al., "Can Soft Drink Taxes Reduce Population Weight?" *Contemp. Econ. Policy* 28 (2010): 23–35.

34 J. P. Block et al., "Point-of-Purchase Price and Education Intervention to Reduce Consumption of Sugary Soft Drinks," *Am. J. Public Health* 100 (2010): 1427–33.

35 J. L. Pomeranz, "Advanced Policy Options to Regulate Sugar-Sweetened Beverages to Support Public Health," *J. Public Health Policy* 33 (2012): 75–88.

36 J. F. Chriqui et al., "State Sales Tax Rates for Soft Drinks and Snacks Sold Through Grocery Stores and Vending Machines, 2007," *J. Public Health Policy* 29 (2008): 226–49.

37 M. L. Kolsgaard et al., "Ethnic Differences in Metabolic Syndrome Among Overweight and Obese Children and Adolescents: The Oslo Adiposity Intervention Study," *Acta Paediatr.* 97 (2008): 1557–63.

38 Y. C. Wang et al., "A Penny-per-Ounce Tax on Sugar-Sweetened Beverages Would Cut Health and Cost Burdens of Diabetes," *Health Affair.* 31 (2012): 199–207.

39 R. Sturm et al., "Soda Taxes, Soft Drink Consumption, and Children's Body Mass Index," *Health Affair.* 29 (2010): 1052–58.

40 R. H. Lustig et al., "The Toxic Truth About Sugar," *Nature* 487 (2012): 27–29.

41   P. J. Gruenewald et al., "Evaluating the Alcohol Environment: Community
      Geography and Alcohol Problems," *Alcohol Res. Health* 26 (2002): 42–48.
42   W. Gosliner et al., "Would Students Prefer to Eat Healthier Foods at School?" *J.
      School Health* 81 (2011): 146–51.
43   M. Moss, "Philadelphia School Battles Students' Bad Eating Habits, on Campus
      and Off," *New York Times* March 27, 2011, www.nytimes.com/2011/03/28/
      us/28food.html?_r=3&pagewanted=2.
44   Wikinvest. Corn. http://www.wikinvest.com/commodity/Corn.
45   J. M. Alston et al., "Farm Subsidies and Obesity in the United States," University
      of California, Berkeley, 2007, giannini.ucop.edu/media/are-update/files/articles/
      v11n2_1.pdf.
46   Food and Water Watch et al., "Do Farm Subsidies Cause Obesity? Dispelling
      Common Myths About Public Health and the Farm Bill," Robert Wood Johnson
      Foundation, 2011, www.foodandwaterwatch.org/tools-and-resources/do-farm-
      subsidies-cause-obesity/.
47   Interview with Ted Miguel, economist at University of California–Berkeley, at
      www.gatesfoundation.org/global-development/Pages/ted-miguel-interview-
      water-sanitation-hygiene.aspx.

Epilogue

1   M. S. Wertz et al., "The Toxic Effects of Cigarette Additives, Philip Morris'
      Project Mix Reconsidered: An Analysis of Documents Released Through
      Litigation," *PLoS Med.* (December 8, 2011): e1001145.

GLOSSARY

ALT: alanine aminotransferase—a blood test that tells about liver function, and is very sensitive to the amount of fat in the liver

Amygdala: the area of the brain that generates the feeling of fear and stress, and causes the body to make extra cortisol

Autonomic nervous system: that part of the nervous system that controls unconscious functions of the body; the sympathetic system controls heart rate, blood pressure, and temperature; while the parasympathetic system controls eating, digestion, and absorption—the two together control energy balance

Cortisol: the stress hormone that acutely mobilizes sugar for use, but that chronically lays down visceral fat

Developmental programming: alterations in brain or body functioning due to alterations in the environment that occur in the fetus prior to birth

Dopamine: a neurotransmitter that when released acutely can cause feelings of reward, but when released chronically reduces its effect, leading to tolerance

Dopamine D_2 receptor: the protein that binds dopamine to generate the reward signal, and that is reduced in density to lead to tolerance

Endocannabinoid: a neurotransmitter that binds to brain receptors and acts like marijuana, driving reward

Enteral: entering the body via the mouth

Epigenetics: modifications in DNA without changes in the DNA genetic sequence, usually occurring prior to birth

Estrogen: female sex hormone, made either in the ovary or in fat tissue

Ghrelin: a hormone made by the stomach that conveys a signal of hunger to the hypothalamus

Hypothalamus: the area at the base of the brain that controls hormone release from various glands

Insulin: the hormone that tells the liver to store glycogen, the fat cells to store energy, and interferes with the leptin signal to increase food intake

Insulin resistance: the state where insulin signaling is reduced, requiring the beta-cells of the pancreas to make more insulin

Insulin secretion: the process of insulin release in response to both rising blood glucose and the firing of the vagus nerve

Leptin: a hormone released from fat cells that travels in the bloodstream to the hypothalamus to report on peripheral energy stores

Leptin resistance: the state where the leptin signal is dampened, leading to the hypothalamus interpreting starvation

Maillard reaction: the binding of a simple sugar (glucose or fructose) to a protein, making the protein less flexible, and generating reactive oxygen species in the process

Metabolic syndrome: a cluster of chronic metabolic diseases characterized by energy overload of the mitochondria

Micronutrient: vitamins or minerals found in real food, usually isolated with the fiber fraction

Mitochondria: areas within the cell that burn either fat or carbohydrate for energy

Neurotransmitter: a chemical in the brain, made in one nerve cell, that when released causes other nerve cells to fire

Nucleus accumbens (NA): the area of the brain that receives the dopamine signal and interprets this as reward

Obesity: excess body fat deposition

Obesogen: a chemical that increases the amount of fat stored, to a greater extent than the calories released when it is burned

Octreotide: a drug similar to the hormone somatostatin that suppresses numerous hormones in the body, especially growth hormone and insulin

Parenteral: entering the body via injection, as into a muscle or vein

Peptide YY$_{(3-36)}$: a hormone made by the small intestine, in response to food, that signals satiety to the hypothalamus

Peroxisome: an area of the cell that contains antioxidants to detoxify reactive oxygen species

Reactive oxygen species: chemicals generated from cellular metabolism that can cause protein or lipid damage, and can lead to cell dysfunction or death if not detoxified by antioxidants

Satiety: the feeling of fullness, mediated by PYY$_{(3-36)}$ action in the hypothalamus

Subcutaneous fat: the fat outside of the abdomen, which is a storehouse of extra energy but does not signify an increased risk for metabolic syndrome

Sympathetic nervous system: that part of the autonomic nervous system that raises heart rate, increases blood pressure, and burns energy

Tolerance: the state where the signal for reward is dampened and can be generated only with the consumption of more substrate (in the case of obesity, palatable food)

Transcription factor: a protein in cells that turns on genes to make the cells change their function

Type 1 diabetes: a disease of high blood sugar due to inadequate insulin production by the beta-cells of the pancreas

Type 2 diabetes: a disease of high blood sugar due to defective insulin action on tissues

Vagus nerve: that part of the autonomic nervous system that promotes food digestion, absorption, and energy storage

Ventral tegmental area (VTA): the area of the brain that sends the dopamine signal signifying reward to the nucleus accumbens

Ventromedial hypothalamus (VMH): the area of the hypothalamus that receives hormonal information from the body to regulate energy balance

Visceral fat: the fat around the organs in the abdomen that is a risk factor for diabetes, heart disease, and stroke, and a marker for metabolic syndrome

INDEX